Dancing for Their Lives

Global Perspectives on Aging

Series editor, Sarah Lamb

This series publishes books that will deepen and expand our understanding of age, aging, ageism, and late life in the United States and beyond. The series focuses on anthropology while being open to ethnographically vivid and theoretically rich scholarship in related fields, including sociology, religion, cultural studies, social medicine, medical humanities, gender and sexuality studies, human development, critical and cultural gerontology, and age studies. Books will be aimed at students, scholars, and occasionally the general public.

Jason Danely, *Aging and Loss: Mourning and Maturity in Contemporary Japan*
Parin Dossa and Cati Coe, eds., *Transnational Aging and Reconfigurations of Kin Work*
Sarah Lamb, ed., *Successful Aging as a Contemporary Obsession: Global Perspectives*
Margaret Morganroth Gullette, *Ending Ageism, or How Not to Shoot Old People*
Ellyn Lem, *Gray Matters: Finding Meaning in the Stories of Later Life*
Michele Ruth Gamburd, *Linked Lives: Elder Care, Migration, and Kinship in Sri Lanka*
Yohko Tsuji, *Through Japanese Eyes: Thirty Years of Studying Aging in America*
Jessica C. Robbins, *Aging Nationally in Contemporary Poland: Memory, Kinship, and Personhood*
Rose K. Keimig, *Growing Old in a New China: Transitions in Elder Care*
Anna I. Corwin, *Embracing Age: How Catholic Nuns Became Models of Aging Well*
Molly George, *Aging in a Changing World: Older New Zealanders and Contemporary Multiculturalism*
Cati Coe, *Changes in Care: Aging, Migration, and Social Class in West Africa*
Megha Amrith, Victoria K. Sakti, and Dora Sampaio, eds., *Aspiring in Later Life: Movements across Time, Space, and Generations*
Cristina Douglas and Andrew Whitehouse, eds., *More-than-Human Aging: Animals, Robots, and Care in Later Life*
Casey Golomski, *God's Waiting Room: Racial Reckoning at Life's End*
Claudia Huang, *Dancing for Their Lives: The Pursuit of Meaningful Aging in Urban China*

Dancing for Their Lives

The Pursuit of Meaningful Aging in Urban China

CLAUDIA HUANG

Rutgers University Press
New Brunswick, Camden, and Newark, New Jersey
London and Oxford

Rutgers University Press is a department of Rutgers, The State University of New Jersey, one of the leading public research universities in the nation. By publishing worldwide, it furthers the University's mission of dedication to excellence in teaching, scholarship, research, and clinical care.

Library of Congress Cataloging-in-Publication Data

Names: Huang, Claudia, author.
Title: Dancing for their lives : the pursuit of meaningful aging in urban China / Claudia Huang.
Description: New Brunswick, New Jersey : Rutgers University Press, 2025. | Series: Global perspectives on aging | Includes bibliographical references and index.
Identifiers: LCCN 2024016369 | ISBN 9781978838871 (paperback) | ISBN 9781978838888 (hardcover) | ISBN 9781978838895 (epub) | ISBN 9781978838901 (pdf)
Subjects: LCSH: Population aging—Social aspects—China—Chengdu. | Older women. | Dance—Social aspects—China—Chengdu. | Resilience (Personality trait)—China—Chengdu.
Classification: LCC HQ1064.C6 H836 2025 | DDC 306.4/846095138—dc23/eng/20240814
LC record available at https://lccn.loc.gov/2024016369

A British Cataloging-in-Publication record for this book is available from the British Library.
Copyright © 2025 by Claudia Huang
All rights reserved

No part of this book may be reproduced or utilized in any form or by any means, electronic or mechanical, or by any information storage and retrieval system, without written permission from the publisher. Please contact Rutgers University Press, 106 Somerset Street, New Brunswick, NJ 08901. The only exception to this prohibition is "fair use" as defined by U.S. copyright law.

References to internet websites (URLs) were accurate at the time of writing. Neither the author nor Rutgers University Press is responsible for URLs that may have expired or changed since the manuscript was prepared.

⊖ The paper used in this publication meets the requirements of the American National Standard for Information Sciences—Permanence of Paper for Printed Library Materials, ANSI Z39.48-1992.

rutgersuniversitypress.org

For my parents and their generation

Contents

	Preface and Acknowledgments	ix
	Introduction: The Age of Uncertainty	1
1	Dancing for Their Lives	19
2	*Dama* Mania	37
3	Families under (Peer) Pressure	54
4	Play a Day, Count a Day	73
5	The Flavor of Life	91
	Conclusion	115
	References	127
	Index	135

Preface and Acknowledgments

I can still remember the look of deep skepticism and amusement that washed over Teacher Yuan's face the first time she saw me dance. Ethnographic research relies on trust, and I am grateful that Teacher Yuan, as well as scores of other "dancing grannies" in Chengdu, overcame their skepticism and trusted me to be a part of their lives for nearly two years. Teacher Yuan never ceased to be amused by my lack of grace, but she and the other women I spent time with were consistently welcoming and patient with my questions and intrusions. They were interested and invested in my research in ways I didn't expect: people often sent me links to relevant news stories or blog posts, sought me out to relate events or stories they thought I would find interesting, or put me in touch with their friends for additional perspectives. I believe they were willing to share so much with me because they understood—certainly more than I did at the beginning—that they were taking part in more than just a massive social dance phenomenon. The story of congregational dancing is also a story about growing older during uncertain times, a subject that is not necessarily universal in its appeal but relatable to anyone who hopes to live a long life. And, though I'm still not much of a dancer these days, I credit them for making me appreciate it in ways I never did before.

Doing research in the People's Republic of China can be a frustrating business. One encounters certain kinds of bureaucratic violence that is impossible to avoid and difficult to convey after the fact. These conditions have only worsened in more recent years. Yet whenever I think back on the time I spent in Chengdu conducting fieldwork, I am struck again and again by the incredible kindness I received from both those who were charged to help me (by professional or social obligation) and from complete strangers. Family and friends hosted me for countless meals. Professor He Mingjie and other faculty and students of the sociology department at Sichuan University encouraged my research and asked clarifying questions. Local government officials and community social workers spoke to me candidly despite being incredibly busy and at times confused about the nature of my project. There were countless people who generously gave of themselves, their resources, and their time. I am thankful to each and every one of them even though most remain unnamed in this book.

I also feel very fortunate to have been surrounded by dedicated mentors and supportive colleagues during my graduate studies, when this project began, and in the years since. My advisor and dissertation committee chair Yunxiang Yan has been a steadfast model of hard work, intellectual curiosity, and self-discipline. From the first time we met, Dr. Yan was a source of both scholarly and personal inspiration for me. Being his student has made me a better anthropologist and a better human. I am grateful to Nancy Levine for always pushing my writing to its fullest potential, and for the warmth and friendship she has extended to me over the years. I cannot count how many hours I spent sitting in her office or her backyard discussing everything from anthropological theory to Los Angeles restaurants; these conversations are among the fondest memories I have from graduate school. Mariko Tamanoi was a constant voice of encouragement throughout my studies; I hope I can emulate her graciousness and kindness in my own career. I am thankful for Andrea Goldman, who reminded me to take a longer view of Chinese history. My work has benefited immensely from her guidance. I also owe a debt of gratitude to Jennifer Jackson, who passed away in 2015. Though I was her student for a few short years before her untimely death, Jennifer's wisdom and generosity continue to guide me to this day.

Like most books based on dissertations, this book has undergone many rounds of revisions. I made the majority of these changes during my time as An Wang postdoctoral fellow at Harvard University's Fairbank Center for Chinese Studies. The Fairbank Center was a nourishing intellectual home. I owe the subtitle of this book—and the concept of "meaningful aging"—to Arthur Kleinman and Winnie Yip, my two mentors during the fellowship, along with the brilliant thinkers who were part of our Meaningful Aging in China discussion group. I found their collective knowledge and commitment to be deeply inspiring and hope that this book does justice to some of the ideas we shared.

Since this book grapples with the ways in which social change impacts aging, I'm honored that it appears alongside many superb works of scholarship in the Global Perspectives on Aging series by Rutgers University Press. Its inclusion in this series would not have been possible without the series editor Sarah Lamb, who not only saw the potential in my work and gave me feedback on the manuscript but also shared her wisdom about each step of the revision and submission process. I have had the great fortune of working with Kimberly Guinta, Carah Naseem, Emma-Li Downer, and the rest of the editorial team at RUP. As a first-time author, I very much appreciated their professionalism and patience.

My name appears alone in the byline of this book, but I have been helped along the way by many others. Some of my friends have read so many drafts and iterations that they must be nearly as relieved at its publication as I am. Annie Malcolm, Megan Steffen, Kathryn Cai, Cari Merritt, Jananie Kalyanamaran, Yael Assor, Anoush Suni, Gwyneth Talley, Eva Melstrom, Erin Thomason, and many others gave me much of their time, insight, and encouragement during the writing and revision process. They pushed me to deepen my thinking, clarify my writing, and above all remain faithful to my own voice. I'm also grateful to my former student assistants from the CSULB Department of Human Development, Maritza Ramirez and Trina Hoang, for reading the entire manuscript from start to finish and helping me reorganize the chapters. There are many additional people I have not named here who have provided indispensable support: colleagues who shared ideas at conferences, mentors who have offered informal feedback, and the three anonymous peer reviewers who provided incredibly helpful feedback. I thank them for being in dialogue with me and look forward to continuing the conversation.

Different phases of this project were generously supported by the Fulbright-Hays Dissertation Research Fellowship, the Harvard University Fairbank Center for Chinese Studies, CSULB College of Liberal Arts, the UCLA Graduate Student Mentorship, the UCLA Dissertation Year Fellowship, the UCLA Center for Chinese Studies, the Duthie-Secchia research award, the UCLA International Institute, the UCLA Urban Humanities Initiative, and the UCLA Department of Anthropology. An earlier version of chapter 2 was previously published in the *Journal of Aging Studies,* and an earlier version of chapter 3 was previously published in *Chinese Families Upside Down,* a collection of essays edited by Yunxiang Yan.

Last but not least, I cannot fully express how grateful I am to the close friends and family whom I have leaned on for the duration of this project. My husband, Noah, stayed up late with me on many nights to keep me company and listen to me read paragraphs aloud. My friend Kendell Sadiik offered humor, sage advice, and twenty-minute dinner recipes when I hit rough patches. Michelle Gomez, Gley Rodriguez, and the teachers at the Isabel Patterson Center for Child Development doted on my child while I worked. Finally, I must acknowledge my parents, who gave up the security and comfort of a life they knew well so that I can live mine with more freedom and possibility. Thank you.

Dancing for Their Lives

Introduction

•••••••••••••••••••

The Age of Uncertainty

> 老娘在外面扳命，老头在里面等死
>
> *Old women are outside struggling for their lives, old men are inside waiting to die.*
> —Local saying in Chengdu

In 2020, a fifty-six-year-old retired Chinese woman named Su Min became an internet sensation when she left her abusive marriage to experience the freedom of the open road. She explained her rationale for making this dramatic change on a personal blog post: "The first half of my life was mainly about enduring," she wrote. "I was a wife, a mother, and a grandmother. One day, I made up my mind to live for myself."

According to various interviews she gave to media outlets, Su Min grew up with domineering parents in a small, remote village in Tibet where her father was posted for work. The village offered few playmates. Her dreams of seeing the world were met with mockery and derision by her family, and she was forced to become a caretaker to her two younger brothers at an early age. When she was eighteen, Su Min's father was transferred back to a work unit in the family's hometown in Henan, a landlocked province in central China. The whole family uprooted with him. Now an adult, Su Min was assigned a job in the same fertilizer factory where her father was a lab director. She toiled at the factory by day and continued to care for her brothers at night.

Desperate to make a life for herself, Su Min married a man despite having only met him twice. It didn't turn out the way she hoped. In another blog post written shortly after she began her road trip, Su Min likened the transition from her parents' house to her marital home to "going from one tunnel into another—dim, silent, and depressing." Her husband was critical and controlling, and the abuse escalated when the fertilizer factory shut down and Su Min lost her job. The fact that she was one of millions of workers who became unemployed due to nationwide economic reforms did not stop him from treating the situation as Su Min's personal failure.

Still, Su Min stayed in the marriage so that her daughter could grow up in a stable home. The country changed in the meantime: small villages became burgeoning metropolises, customs and traditions shifted, and people began to want new and different things. Su Min's daughter eventually went to college and married a classmate. With two white-collar jobs in expanding fields, the young couple was on track to have much higher wages and a better quality of life compared to their parents. Eager to do as much as possible to assist them on this life trajectory, Su Min dutifully became a full-time caregiver again when she became a grandmother to twin boys. While her daughter and son-in-law hustled to stay afloat in the increasingly competitive economy, Su Min fed, changed, bathed, and played with the babies.

Yet the years of persistent toil and hardship did not dampen her urge to escape her confined world. At some point, she came across an online article about cross-country car camping and decided to make her dream a reality. As her grandsons grew up and entered preschool, Su Min took on multiple jobs—in a supermarket, as a street cleaner, for a delivery service—to save up to buy a used car. She also began to research driving routes and purchase camping equipment. Finally, on September 23, 2020, she drove out of the underground garage at her apartment complex and watched her daughter slowly disappear in the rearview mirror.

"The hardest parts of life are in the past," she wrote in a blog post reflecting on her frame of mind at this pivotal moment. "I had a baby, I raised my daughter into adulthood, I watched her get married and have her own children, I raised those grandchildren until they were old enough to go to school. I have fulfilled all the social obligations of motherhood. After I turned fifty, I stopped menstruating, memory loss and wrinkles rushed into life at an accelerated rate. I felt I couldn't wait any longer. This time, I am certain that nothing—not age, marriage, money, or family—can stop me. I am leaving at this moment no matter what."

Finding Meaning in Between

This book is about Chinese women of Su Min's generation and their pursuit of personal meaning as they age. It is about the entanglements between personal and national transformation. Most of all, it is about the ways in which social circumstances can change the way that people grow older, and conversely how people's private revelations about the aging process can rend and reshape the social fabric.

Su Min's story caught my attention when it went viral on Chinese social media because it echoed so much of my research on retired women who participate in what I call the "congregational dancing" phenomenon (Huang 2016). Congregational dance groups—popularly known as "dancing grannies"—are nothing short of a cultural and media sensation in China. Anyone who has traveled to a Chinese city in the past fifteen years will be familiar with the sight and sound of groups of middle-aged and older women (as well as a few men) dancing together in public areas. They appear in the early morning hours in parks, public plazas, riverbanks, and commercial squares with their portable speakers to dance the morning away. They appear again in the evenings, filling the air with the sound of upbeat music, laughter, and revelry. There are an estimated one hundred million such dancers scattered throughout China. This is a staggering figure. To put it into context, it is roughly a third of the population of the entire United States and 7 percent of the total Chinese population. When I first started seeing these groups appear on once-quiet street corners in the late 2000s during my annual visits, I began to wonder who these people were, what they wanted, and why they were dancing.

Bitter as it was, Su Min's story is far from unusual. Throughout the course of my research, I encountered hundreds of women whose pasts resembled hers: they were born in the years and decades immediately following the Communist takeover in 1949, endured the political turmoil of the Cultural Revolution in their childhoods, spent their youths undergoing forced "reeducation" in rural areas, were limited to having a single child by the one-child policy, and then were laid off from their jobs during the country's stunning transformation into the world's second-largest economy. Even for those who kept their jobs during this period of economic transition, their eventual retirement likely was not a matter of personal choice due to mandatory retirement ages. In China, people in this age cohort are sometimes referred to as the "lost generation" because their lives were repeatedly upended by the social and political turmoil of the second half of the twentieth century. They have an unusually strong generational identity: women of this generation are called *dama*—literally meaning "big mother"—a term that signifies a certain shared appearance, comportment, and set of interests. For many of them, retirement is the first time they have ever lived outside of direct state control. Their determination to make the most of their newfound freedom—all the while navigating contracting social safety nets and increasingly youth-oriented cultural values—is the central story of this book.

When I began asking questions about the congregational dancing phenomenon in conversation with friends and family, people offered plenty of theories about why so many older women were dancing in the streets. These explanations tended to focus on what the *dama* lack: They dance because they lost their jobs and have nothing else to do. They dance because they grew up in a collectivist society and cannot adapt to more modern, more individualistic times. They dance because they're not young anymore but don't want to feel invisible. All of these narratives have threads of truth in them. I found, however, that congregational dancers themselves overwhelmingly explain their participation not in terms of what is missing from life but rather what it still has to offer. As one woman told me, "Some of us haven't worked since our forties. But life doesn't end there! We still have energy to spend, and it has to go somewhere. So we come and we dance, and we live our lives with a little flavor." What exactly she means by "flavor" will be the focus of a later chapter, but for now, it suffices to say that retired women join dance groups because they want to live with meaning and purpose.

In many ways, congregational dance groups are unlikely venues for meaning-making to take place. They serve no overt higher function and exist purely for the enjoyment of their participants. Virtually no groups engage in choreography, and some of the dancing can appear uninspired or uncreative. Though most groups practice weekly or even daily, there is no explicit goal that they are working toward—no big performance, no standard of achievement, no final recital. They just show up at the same place, at the same time, with the same people, and dance. Many Chinese urbanites I spoke to characterized the congregational dancing phenomenon as fundamentally unserious. It is either the accidental byproduct of historical events without weight or substance its own, or else just a bunch of retirees "playing around," or more derisively, "wasting time." I think this interpretation is inaccurate. At the same time, I acknowledge that my own argument—that *dama* are trying to make sense of their lives with a feverish urgency by devoting themselves to leisure and fun—sounds a bit like a contradiction in terms.

And yet, there is nothing new or surprising about this paradox at the heart of the phenomenon. The pursuit of meaning is a complicated endeavor in an authoritarian society. During the decades of Mao Zedong's autocratic rule, Chinese urbanites were expected to sacrifice their individual aspirations and desires in exchange for a wide social safety net that included guaranteed jobs, housing, health care, and education (Tang and Parish 2000). The reform era ushered in a new kind of social contract that allows for individual expression in private realms but still very much regulates it in matters of public interest—a set of conditions that Li Zhang and Aihwa Ong (2008) have identified as "socialism from afar." Many avenues that people elsewhere may take to give their lives purpose—political activism, civic engagement, and religious practice—are either tightly controlled or banned altogether in China. For people who are excluded from the workforce but in search of a meaningful community, congregational dance groups are perhaps the only widely available option. Their perceived vapidness, in other words, is their superpower.

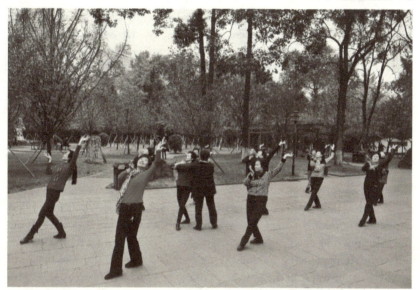

FIGURE 1 A congregational dance group practicing in a Chengdu park while a hired dance teacher makes adjustments. (Photo by Claudia Huang)

In *Everything Was Forever, Until It Was No More,* his aptly titled book about the final years of the Soviet Union, Alexei Yurchak (2005) writes that a new style of living that straddled the line between "inside" and "outside" the authoritarian system emerged during late socialism. It came about from a deep sense of cynicism about the official Soviet ideology, which had become utterly detached from reality by the 1970s. While people went through the performative motions of praising socialist values (sometimes even marching with official signs without caring about what was written on them), they privately had no faith in these values or the government that promoted them. Many were also turned off by the strident sincerity of the dissident movement. Instead, they preferred to try to live outside of politics altogether by participating in informal clubs and interest groups. Called "being *vyne*," or "living outside," these new lifestyles "generated multiple new temporalities, spatialities, social relations, and meanings that were not necessarily anticipated or controlled by the state, although they were fully made possible by it." To put it another way, Yurchak's work seeks to dispel the notion that people living under authoritarian regimes can be neatly divided into "dissidents" and "accomplices," and argues that there is no "objective" reality other than the one people and governments co-construct through everyday discourses.

"Being *vyne*" serves as a helpful road map for thinking through how retired women in China pursue meaningful aging by playing around with their friends.

In a society where political ideology dominates public discourse about what matters in life, there is little space to explore questions of identity and values in the open. Instead, these conversations must take place obliquely, nonconfrontationally, and in the spaces in between. Dancing, socializing, and leisure take on a new kind of significance when seen in this light.

Retired women's efforts to live on their own terms may not be revolutionary, but they are still rebellious acts that challenge normative social values. Su Min told a reporter that just before she left for her first road trip, her husband had asked her, "What will happen if every Chinese woman is as selfish as you?" His attitude isn't out of the ordinary: while there are people who believe that women's post-retirement self-cultivation activities—chief among them congregational dancing—have made a positive contribution to society, I found that the default opinion among Chinese urbanites fell somewhere between grudging tolerance and downright contempt. The sheer number of retired women out in the streets dancing and socializing demonstrates that the *dama* have not let this disapproval stop them. In response to her husband's question, Su Min reportedly told him, "Then they'll be just as happy as I am."

Meaningful Aging

None of what I describe in this book would have been possible even one generation ago. Su Min set off on her road trip and millions of women joined congregational dance groups when they reached late middle age because there has been a sea change in how old age is perceived and practiced in China today. People who experienced the brunt of the radical social changes of the past half-century are now growing older in a historical moment where the cultural frameworks that once supported old age are in flux. China is now the fastest-aging nation in the world. By the Chinese state's own projections, people over age sixty-five will outnumber those under fourteen by 2030. Even more alarmingly, some demographers predict that over a quarter of China's population will be over sixty-five by the year 2050. That's roughly five hundred million people. It is difficult to overstate the potential ramifications of this aging trend for China's continued economic expansion, for its already precarious social harmony, and even for its national security.

Because China became an aging society over the course of just a single generation, it offers an incisive look at the ways in which demographic shifts can exert pressure on cultural processes. While much has been written on China's aging population from the vantages of eldercare and institutional reforms—often with a focus on older adults' struggles to cope with forces beyond their control—how old age is understood and practiced by the rising generation of Chinese elders is a story that remains largely untold. Their dogged perseverance in these efforts demonstrates that older adults are not merely adapting to a changing world; they are actively creating new shared aesthetics, modes of social connection, and value systems. By forging new ways to grow old, retired women in urban China are living proof that old age can be a potent site for social production.

Like millions of others around the globe who grew up in the middle of the twentieth century, Chinese retirees are growing old in a world that barely resembles the one in which they were born. For them, the aging process comes with novel challenges and burdens. It also offers tremendous opportunity to renegotiate relationships, cultivate new interests and connections, and seek personal fulfillment on their own terms. Though I focus on the plight of Chinese retirees in this book, the question of meaningful aging has global implications. We are living in a rapidly aging world. According to the World Health Organization (WHO), the number of people aged sixty and above will double to 2.1 billion by 2050, and the number of people over eighty will triple to 426 million in that same time frame (WHO 2022). Already, the macro-level economic and social ramifications of this demographic transition are playing out around the globe: from broad protests against retirement age reform in France to shrinking economic growth due to the declining working-age population in Japan, aging populations present a myriad of challenges and opportunities for societies on every continent. Nordic countries, for example, started paying attention to population aging as early as the 1940s, and China's neighbor Japan has also been contending with a remarkably top-heavy population since the mid- to late twentieth century.

New demographic realities have brought about new ways of thinking about old age as well as new expectations about the role that older people ought to play in society. In the United States, significant shifts in social policy and cultural discourse on aging began to emerge in the 1970s and 1980s when post–World War II birth rates began to decline and the baby boomer generation approached middle age. In *Why Survive,* the Pulitzer Prize–winning book published in 1975 detailing the "tragic" state of old age in America, psychiatrist Robert Butler argues that having the ability to survive into old age is meaningless unless people can actually enjoy these "extra" years. Butler, who is often dubbed the "father of modern gerontology," not only coined the term "ageism" to describe the stigma experienced by older adults, but also promoted "productive aging"—an approach to growing old that emphasizes elders' continued participation in the workforce (Butler and Gleason 1985).

This line of thinking gained even more traction when physician John Rowe and psychologist Robert Kahn created a model of "successful aging." Like Butler's thesis on age, Rowe and Kahn's ideas emerged during a period of American history marked by contracting social safety nets and an increasingly neoliberal governance framework. But Butler was mostly concerned with laws and policies affecting older adults, whereas Rowe and Kahn focused their attentions on personal agency. In their widely read book, they encourage older adults to take charge of their own aging by avoiding disease, maintaining cognitive and physical function, and remaining engaged in their communities (Rowe and Kahn 1997). Their message resonated. The "successful aging" movement, as it came to be called, garnered enormous influence in both scholarly and popular discourses throughout the world. While the ostensible goal of the movement is to empower older adults, its emphasis on productivity and individual autonomy can be counterproductive. In her critique of the successful aging paradigm, Sarah Lamb (2013) notes that people who aspire to age "successfully" under Rowe and Kahn's model think of themselves as projects that can be continuously improved and can feel like failures if they become ill or experience the normal declines that come with growing older.

Though I never heard anyone mentioning Rowe and Kahn by name, the successful aging paradigm has certainly taken root in China. In their efforts to address the rapidly aging population and an oncoming eldercare crisis, both local and central government officials make regular references to the need for elders to take responsibility for their own health and well-being. The term used most frequently in Chinese gerontological circles and spaces is *jiji yanglao*, or "active aging." The congregational dancing phenomenon is sometimes held up in promotional materials as an example of *jiji yanglao*, where it is primarily depicted as a form of low-impact aerobic exercise suitable for seniors. While some *dama* I met did talk about their participation in terms of wishing to stay healthy and avoiding being a burden on their children, it would be overly simplistic to think of the phenomenon as a Chinese manifestation of the successful aging paradigm. Rather than think of themselves as projects for self-improvement, many *dama* instead engage in self-cultivation. The distinction is subtle but crucial: it is the difference between trying to maintain the ideal of an "ageless self" through work and discipline and trying to discover oneself through a process of open-ended exploration.

In Western social science traditions, the pursuit and cultivation of an individual identity is generally understood to be the province of children and youths. According to psychiatrist and pediatrician Margaret Mahler (1977), individuation-separation is a multiphase process that begins in infancy and concludes in adolescence. The first phase consists of a child learning that she is a separate entity from her mother through the gradual development of independent mobility and mastery of her physical environment. The latter phase happens when an adolescent establishes psychological autonomy from her caregivers, learning to rely on herself for emotional regulation, self-identity, and worldview (Blos 1979). Many of the behaviors associated with teenage rebellion—self-involvement, experimentation, questioning or flouting social norms, seeking approval from peers rather than family—occur during this time.

The period of individuation and separation is thought to occur in early life because it is what has been observed, and because these observations confirm scholarly theories. I have no bone to pick with the field of developmental psychology, nor do I deny that young people from the countries where many scholars hail do tend to establish a fuller sense of self during adolescence. The conventional wisdom about teenage behavior is so deeply entrenched in the popular imagination because it is so frequently reflected by reality. The fact remains, however, that I have observed something different in urban China. There, a major developmental leap appears to take place in the years immediately following retirement, and it is retirees who are trying out new pastimes, pursuing new dreams, and reimagining identities distinct from those expected by their families. It is plausible, then, that historical and cultural circumstances produced the adolescent behaviors observed by Western psychologists. Under different conditions, is it not also possible that these same behaviors can be observed in people at a different point in the life course?

To illustrate my point, it is worthwhile to first revisit the historical circumstances that gave rise to adolescence as we know it today. In the United States, the links between the emergence of the "teenage years" and social-economic circumstances have been well-documented by social scientists of multiple disciplines. In the early twentieth century and especially in the postwar period, American adolescents gained an unprecedented amount of free time because the forces of industrialization, urbanization, and economic expansion meant that many families no longer relied on their children's labor—and adolescents became consumers in their own right. During their newfound free time, these youths experimented with new musical genres like rock 'n' roll and aesthetic genres like "greaser" culture. They pushed social norms, engaged in premarital sexual relationships, and forced advertisers to pay heed to their preferences due to their increased spending power. In other words, they took part in building the foundations of a youth culture that arguably transformed the social fabric of the latter half of the twentieth century. But just as this life stage arose during a time of dramatic social and economic transformation, major shifts in the underpinnings of Chinese society have also paved the way for the appearance of a new way of inhabiting a time of life. A big difference, in this case, is that it is early old age, rather than early adulthood, that is in the midst of becoming something new.

Examining the congregational dancing phenomenon from a generational or developmental cohort perspective can help clarify a seeming contradiction. On the one hand, it is clearly an example of what Yunxiang Yan (2009) has termed the individualization of Chinese society. After being unwillingly liberated from the security of state-organized professional and social lives, people joined dance groups in order to focus on themselves and their own interests.

On the other hand, they are doing so by participating in a massive social phenomenon. Falling in line is part of the essence of congregational dancing. The women who participate literally wear the same outfits, listen to the same music, and do the same moves as millions of other people. However, conformity and self-cultivation are not necessarily incompatible goals given the cultural and historical context. Because the social distortions of the twentieth century disproportionately affected one particular cohort, this cohort was tasked not only with redefining their individual selves but also reinventing a generational identity.

The emergence of "teenagers" in the United States and the emergence of *dama* in China have a lot of parallels. Both were brought about by massive economic restructuring that afforded free time to a generation of people who otherwise would have been engaged in labor. In both cases, a generational cohort gave rise to a highly visible subculture that challenged preexisting social conventions. Finally, in both cases, adherents to the new subculture place a premium on personal expression and exploring new possibilities heretofore off-limits to them by virtue of their positions in their respective societies. There is one important difference: while teens in postwar America had the benefit of youth, Chinese *dama*'s advanced age gives their pursuit of personal meaning a deeper sense of urgency. To put it another way, this generation of Chinese women is dancing for their lives.

What about Men?

This book focuses almost exclusively on the lives and experiences of retired urban women. The reasons for this are primarily practical: though there are a small number of men who participate in the dance groups—particularly in groups that practice ballroom or Latin dance styles where people ideally dance in opposite-gendered pairs—the vast majority of congregational dancers are women between the ages of fifty-five and seventy-five. This gender imbalance can be explained by a number of factors, the most significant being the gender difference in compulsory retirement age. With few exceptions, Chinese men are compelled to retire at sixty. Women must retire even earlier: the retirement age is fifty-five for women in white-collar careers and fifty for women in blue-collar careers. Moreover, many women who participate in dance groups did not retire when they reached official retirement age but were instead cast out of the work force at even younger ages when China launched state-owned enterprise (SOE) reforms in the late 1990s and early 2000s. Women, who occupied lower-paying jobs and were assumed to not have as many breadwinning responsibilities as men, were laid off in disproportionate numbers when factories and other SOEs were privatized or closed

(Appleton, Song, and Xia 2005; Ji and Wu 2018). Combined with the fact that women tend to live longer than men, these gender-imbalanced state policies made many urban women "socially old"—in the sense that their retirements curtailed their economic productivity and gave them no choice but to focus on leisure—long before they could be considered older adults in a biological sense.

Nevertheless, retired men certainly exist in large numbers in urban China, and why there has not been a comparable post-retirement phenomenon consisting mostly of older men is somewhat of a mystery. I frequently wondered about retired men during my fieldwork. Where are they? What are they doing? I asked these questions to many people, especially in the early stages of my research. My interlocutors provided a range of explanations: some dance group participants openly bemoaned the fact that their husbands spent most of their time indoors and resisted their wives' efforts to get them to go out more; some younger interlocutors expressed worry about their fathers, whom they noticed were becoming far more idle after retirement when compared to their active mothers. Some retired men I spoke to told me that they had their own hobbies, but that these activities—ranging from photography to day (stock) trading to playing mahjong or Chinese chess—did not require them to be outdoors or visible to the public. Most people referred, at least obliquely, to a popular local Chengdu saying that opens this chapter: "Old women are outside struggling for their lives, old men are inside waiting to die." The expression is meant to be a tongue-in-cheek comment about something widely considered to be common knowledge in Chengdu: retired women typically work hard to stay active and connected, but retired men tend to retreat into isolation once their professional lives are over. There are, of course, people of both genders who undermine these stereotypes, but the generalizations have enough truth in them that the expression has become a cliché. Most people chuckled or smirked when they repeated the saying, but given what we know about the connection between elders' social connections and their physical, mental, and emotional health (see Mor-Barak and Miller 1991; Kawachi and Berkman 2001), the implications of men's comparative lack of post-retirement social engagement for their well-being could be quite serious.

That said, it is beyond the scope of this book to discuss the plight of urban China's retired men, or to explain why women are seemingly participating in collective social enterprises in greater numbers than their male counterparts. I have chosen instead to focus on the first part of the local saying that opens this book: "Old women are outside struggling for their lives." What are the forces they are struggling against? What tools or resources are at their disposal? What is the end goal of their efforts? By highlighting the experiences and inner worlds of middle-aged women, a demographic that has been largely overlooked in both scholarship and popular discourse alike, I seek to demonstrate that their lives can both reflect and refract the social contexts in which they live.

Context of Fieldwork

As governments and institutions attempt to grapple with demographic-driven social turbulence, anthropologists have unique vantage points from which to witness how people experience these broad changes in their everyday lives. Ethnographic inquiry can reveal previously unnoticed patterns and provide insights into the ways in which demographic transitions bring about profound transformations in social networks, intimate relationships, and personal understandings about what it means to grow older.

This book is based on ethnographic research conducted in Chengdu, the capital of Sichuan province in China's southwest. Though it is not particularly well-known internationally, Chengdu has been a culturally and geographically significant place in China for many centuries. It boasts the distinction of being the only major Chinese city that has remained in the same location, and under the same name, for more than two millennia. Sitting in a well-protected plain at the base of the Tibetan plateau and at the intersection of several major trade routes, Chengdu's strategic location has been used by powerful people to their advantage throughout history. The city was the capital of the bronze-age Shu state in the fourth century BC, the capital of the Kingdom of Shu during the Three Kingdoms period (AD 221–263), the capital of a short-lived rebel kingdom led by the peasant leader Zhang Xianzhong from 1643 to1646, and finally as the temporary capital of the embattled Kuomintang government during World War II.

This illustrious history lends the city and its inhabitants a sense of importance and pride, but few people mention these points today when talking about what makes Chengdu unique. Instead, locals might boast about giant pandas, which are native to the surrounding mountains and bred in a well-known research center on the city's outskirts. They might also point you to their favorite places to sample the region's spicy cuisine, which has earned Chengdu a "City of Gastronomy" designation by UNESCO. But Chengdu's main attraction is something less tangible. With its ample green spaces and purportedly the highest number of teahouses per capita in the world, people from all over China come to Chengdu to experience its laid-back attitude, ample opportunities for leisure, and slow pace of life. The city owes much of this reputation to climate and geography. Chengdu, and the fertile basin in which it is situated, has long been called 天府之国, meaning "country of heaven" or "land of abundance." In contrast to other regions in China where agricultural production requires back-breaking work for much of the year, growing food is a little easier on the Chengdu plain, and people living there have long been able to afford to take time to enjoy the finer things in life.

Very few people in modern-day Chengdu still cultivate crops for a living, but the legacy of a leisurely lifestyle has remained. Despite its fourteen million inhabitants, multinational corporations, two international airports, and daily traffic congestion, Chengdu manages to feel quite different from the "first-tier" mega-cities on China's coasts. Its many parks are filled at all hours with people gossiping over a shared bag of sunflower seeds. Shopkeepers regularly doze in their chairs after lunch or abandon their stations altogether to play a card game on the sidewalk with neighbors. After dark, office workers spill out of high-rise buildings and head directly to one of the city's numerous barbecue vendors to enjoy a late-night snack with a cold beer.

Although Chengdu is not the subject of this book, the city's local culture does serve as a backdrop and foundation to the stories I share. I have been asked many times whether I thought the congregational dancing phenomenon is especially popular in Chengdu because its residents are so leisure-focused to begin with. I cannot determine for certain whether there are more dance groups in Chengdu than in other places. The phenomenon enjoys natural advantages in Chengdu compared to hilly cities like nearby Chongqing, which has limited flat space for groups to dance, and compared to northern cities like Beijing or Shenyang, where snowy winters can force groups to take months-long hiatuses. What I can confidently say is that Chengdu's dance groups are numerous, enthusiastic, and seem like a natural feature of the city's preexisting joie de vivre. The importance of relaxation and informal sociality in Chengdu's public culture has been the subject of several works by historian Di Wang (2003, 2008, 2018), who argues that what takes place in Chengdu's teahouses can reveal a lot about urban life in China as a whole. Though this book is not an examination of Chengdu's public culture per se, it is still a portrait of everyday life in the city.

Chengdu is a special place for me. I was born in the Qingyang district near People's Park and lived within a few miles of the city center until I was eight years old. Though we emigrated to the United States and live in California, my parents and I still think of Chengdu as home. My descriptions of the city's landscape, inhabitants, and everyday rhythms were largely recorded during two preliminary trips to the field in the summers of 2014 and 2015 and a year-long period between 2016 and 2017. However, my knowledge of the place has been accumulating for my entire life.

Despite all the ways I am connected to Chengdu and to China, I still hesitate to call this a work of "native" or "insider" anthropology. Proponents of the concept, which has been in circulation since at least the 1970s (Hayano 1979; Narayan 1993; Kanuha 2000), argue that researchers who share cultural and linguistic similarities with the people they study can offer more nuanced accounts than outsiders. But like other ethnographers who were brought up in the liminal space between cultures, I question the usefulness of this dichotomy (see Chawla 2006; Tsuda 2015). Every ethnographer, including ones who have familial or cultural roots in their field sites, brings a unique subject position that informs her perspectives and interpretations.

For me, living in Chengdu as an adult after leaving it as an eight-year-old was an overwhelming experience. I had visited my extended family quite often in the interim years, of course, but I was frequently accompanied by one or both of my parents and treated as a guest by my loving and protective relatives. Staying at either my grandmother or my aunt's home, I was directed on when to wake, where to sit, what and how much to eat, and how often to bathe. What I remember most vividly from those visits is the feeling of having almost no agency whatsoever. My parents often took me along as they embarked on their frenzied quests to reconnect with as many people as possible during our weeks-long visits. I was a passive observer at innumerable tea outings, restaurant dinners, and living room hangouts. If anyone thought it was strange that my parents brought me—at first an awkward teenager and then a young woman—with them on these visits, they did not say so. People offered me hot water, sliced fruit, and life advice, and I politely accepted everything with a smile. No opportunity to explore the city on my own was ever presented, and I seldom sought it out. I honestly cannot say why. Perhaps, because these relatives and family friends never watched me grow up, the dynamic between us was frozen in time and I remained a child in Chengdu despite maturing into adulthood in my American life.

All this is to say that when I arrived in Chengdu as a graduate student with an independent agenda, I encountered a city that was intimately familiar but in some ways also utterly foreign. Along with China as a whole, Chengdu has changed beyond recognition since I was a child. Roughly ten million of its now fourteen million residents moved to the city in the years after I emigrated, and the built environment transformed at such a frenetic pace that my parents and I often got lost during our visits: what was a sleepy neighborhood one year might be a giant shopping center the next. There have also been dizzying technological advancements that can make life in the United States feel positively quaint in comparison. Thanks to the widespread availability of affordable domestically made smartphones, many aspects of urban life—from paying utility bills to purchasing train tickets or making restaurant reservations—are conducted entirely via mobile apps. Even the humblest street vendors selling hand-pulled nougat or knife sharpeners operating out of tricycle carts accept mobile payments by displaying QR code printouts for customers to scan. I devoted considerable time and mental resources to figuring out how to live in a modern Chinese city during my first few months in Chengdu as a researcher. Many of my dance group interlocutors were more tech-savvy than I was despite being several decades older, and I often sought their help with whatever mobile app was stymying me that day.

Of course, looking and sounding like the locals did have its distinct advantages. When conducting observations, my presence was taken for granted, and I never attracted any attention from passersby. I grew up speaking Sichuanese at home with my parents, so I was able to carry out conversations with locals in a shared language. This matters a great deal when conducting research with retirees: though Mandarin is the standard language throughout China and despite the fact that it is nearly universally understood in Han-majority cities, many older adults do not speak it comfortably if they were raised on a different dialect. I conducted all my interviews in Sichuanese. More importantly, I was able to pick up the subtleties in word choice and tone in conversations between my interlocutors while conducting participant observation. My local connections also meant that I was spared some of the brutal loneliness that ethnographic fieldwork is sometimes associated with. I was certainly listless at times, but having a family and friends who could introduce me to people helped my research tremendously, especially in the preliminary stage. I also had the comfort of being able to spend some of my days off in the familiar company of my extended family.

That said, my semi-"insider" status had its pitfalls as well. My blunders and naiveté frequently confused people. When I went to the Sichuan University campus branch of a major Chinese bank to open an account, for example, the incredulous clerk openly voiced his amusement that a twenty-eight-year-old woman did not already have a bank account. International students and foreign scholars of all ages regularly patronize this bank branch, but the clerk did not recognize me—even as I handed him my American passport as identification—as a foreigner. I was seldom afforded the benefit of the doubt that international scholars receive. For instance, when a European friend I had met through the Sichuan University International Students Office decided to join me at a local "old age University" for an exhibition, the gate guards allowed him to pass without incident, while I was escorted upstairs to answer questions about my intentions and show my letter of introduction from my sponsoring department at the university. Many people I spoke to, particularly government officials, expressed surprise or even skepticism about my ignorance of administrative procedures and had to be continually pressed to provide information that they assumed I already knew given my command of the local language.

Neither the perks nor pitfalls associated with my semi-local status changed the fact that I was a young woman trying to understand the experiences of older adults, or the fact that I was a distinctly untalented dancer trying to learn about a social phenomenon centered on bodily movement. I conducted formal and informal interviews with a wide range of people including dance group participants, retirees who participated in other kinds of social groups, government officials, social workers, and eldercare specialists, as well as individuals who simply wanted to share their views about some aspect of my research topic. I also closely analyzed television shows, local periodicals, and internet blogs for insights into how congregational dancing and the plight of China's urban retirees were being interpolated by official and unofficial media sources.

Most of my insights, however, came from conducting participant observation with two dance groups called the "Dancing Beauties" and the "Sunset Dance Group." This meant joining these groups on social outings, group chats on social media, and, of course, dancing along with them during their daily or weekly practices. My interlocutors were overwhelmingly patient and kind with me, but they also made no secret of the fact that they found my physical clumsiness amusing. The full extent of my dance training prior to fieldwork was a few ballet classes in preschool. Despite everyone's overwhelming generosity and patience, I experienced a sharp learning curve when I began dancing. I often made embarrassing mistakes like turning in the wrong direction, missing musical cues, or being out of sync with everyone.

Dancing was not part of my original research plan. When I first began my preliminary research, I observed dozens of groups throughout the city on a rotating basis and asked participants for basic information like how often the group met, whether there was a fee to participate, and whether the participants knew each other prior to joining the group. Whenever possible, I also gathered information about people's employment histories, other post-retirement activities, and why they decided to join a dance group. People were generally happy to answer my questions and often elaborated about these matters or provided additional information (for example, about why they enjoyed dancing) without my asking. It soon became apparent, however, that these methods would be insufficient if I wanted to understand what drew so many retirees to dancing and how the dance groups mediate social connections. I would need to fully participate in the groups if I wanted to go deeper.

Joining the Dancing Beauties and the Sunset Dance Group as a fully participating member offered insights that I could never have obtained had I remained a passive observer. I never mastered any of the dance forms or pieces the groups practiced, but I did improve over time. More importantly, my awkward struggles to dance turned out to be an invaluable source of embodied knowledge, or what dance scholar Barbara Browning (1995) calls "corporeal intelligence." Moreover, fully participating in the group's activities meant that I got to know the other members better and established personal friendships with some of the women. I joined the groups on their social outings, chatted with them on social media, and lingered after dance practices to gossip.

In keeping with the Chinese custom of using kinship terms when addressing people older than oneself in informal social settings, I addressed most of my interlocutors as "Auntie," followed by their surname. A few women preferred to be called by their given names. Over time, many of them also began to refer to me as their "niece" in an affectionate, tongue-in-cheek sort of way. All names that appear in this book are pseudonyms, though I preserved the naming conventions I used while in the field: I substituted given names for given names, and surnames for those I called "Auntie."

Framework of the Book

In chapter 1, I trace the origins of the phenomenon to the economic and demographic shifts that took place in the past half-century. I contend that people seek out dance groups in search of something deeper than exercise and leisure. This chapter showcases how intimate aspects of ordinary people's lives have become entangled with China's national aspirations and explains why so many retired women of this generation searching for sympathy and connection find what they're looking for in dance groups.

Chinese attitudes and practices of aging have changed so much over the past two generations that many retired women feel that they are venturing into uncharted territory as they grow older. In chapter 2, I shed light on how women who participate in congregational dancing became associated with a new category of older person known as *dama*. By examining how social change alters the ways in which people understand and inhabit different stages of the life course, this chapter demonstrates that the *dama* persona constitutes a new gendered aesthetic of aging that responds to a seismic shift in how identity and status are defined in post-reform Chinese society.

Many retired women in China—including those who participate in dance groups—must contend with a fundamental tension in their lives: on the one hand, they are freer than ever before to live their lives on their own terms; on the other hand, expectations that older women devote themselves to their families remain salient in Chinese society and can become especially intense as these women become grandmothers. Chapter 3 examines the uneasy balance that retired women try to strike when confronted with the tension between self-interest and morally laden family obligations in post-reform urban China as well as how friendships figure into this fraught calculus.

Having so far established that older women in urban China lean on each other for self-cultivation opportunities in their present lives, the book in chapter 4 focuses on how they imagine and plan for the future. Because the one-child policy created an upside-down population pyramid, the customary practice of aging at home under the care of an adult child is becoming increasingly untenable. These retirees, in other words, cannot rely on their children to care for them as they grow older. At the same time, the social welfare programs that the government promised in exchange for their reproductive sacrifices never materialized, leaving retirees to plan for old age on their own. This chapter captures the wide range of emotions that retired women have in reaction to this cruel reversal of policy, including bitterness, humor, and denial.

Chapter 5 addresses older adults' quests for meaning. I discuss three attempts that the state has made to regulate the congregational dancing phenomenon and the complex ways that participants have responded to these interventions. Ultimately, the chapter further clarifies the questions that this book seeks to answer: How do people learn to find sweetness and meaning when their lives are overdetermined by forces beyond their control? What exactly does "freedom" mean in an authoritarian state? When everything is subject to government control, what possibilities remain for meaning making?

1
Dancing for Their Lives

● ● ● ● ● ● ● ● ● ● ● ● ● ● ● ● ● ● ● ●

A congregational dancer I call Auntie Deng once offered a particularly poignant summary of her motives for joining a dance group during an interview:

> It used to be that I would wake up, make breakfast for everyone, go to work, pick up my son, prepare dinner for everyone, then supervise my son's schoolwork. But I don't work anymore, and neither does my husband. My son has his own family. If I don't dance, then what do I wake up for? Now, my days go like this: I get up and I come to dance in the mornings. I go home, take a nap, and by the time I get up it's time to make dinner. After dinner [my husband and I] watch TV, then it's time to go to bed again. It takes work to find something to do with all this time! Coming to the dance group gives the day some purpose.

This mundane synopsis of daily life reveals something much deeper: not only have the social-political changes that occurred over the past fifty years changed the Chinese social landscape, but these changes and their consequences have also reshaped the way people relate to their own lived experiences. There are certainly people in China for whom survival and the maintenance of basic living standards is still very much a consideration, but they make up an increasingly small proportion of the population. According to the World Bank, 800 million people have been lifted out of poverty since the initiation of economic reforms in 1978, and "extreme poverty"—defined as living on less than US$1.90 per capita per day, was eradicated by 2021 (World Bank 2023).

For most older people in urban China, the rhythm and demands of daily life bear little resemblance to the lives they were born into and the lives that they perhaps expected to live. What has not changed, however, is the desire to live meaningfully. These days, most retired middle-class urbanites are not concerned about how to put the next meal on the table. What preoccupies them is why they should get up each morning. The broad strokes of this transformation have been depicted by many scholars, and I will not attempt to improve on their efforts here. Instead, I'll let the life history of a woman named Qingyi tell the story.

Living History

Qingyi was born in Chengdu in 1957 as the second child and first daughter of a couple who immigrated to Chengdu from a neighboring province. Her father, a teacher, had been assigned a good job in a vocational school in Chengdu. A younger brother followed a few years after Qingyi was born. Her early childhood was uneventful and pleasant: she spent her days playing with the children of the other teachers and staff members and later attended the primary school attached to the vocational college.

Qingyi was nine years old when the Great Proletarian Cultural Revolution began, sending the country into chaos and upending her insular and peaceful world. Qingyi does not recall the early years of the Cultural Revolution very well, other than the fact that her father's teaching colleagues—sometimes along with their families—disappeared from campus on a regular basis. It was a time of political purges, violent clashes, and widespread paranoia (see Thurston 1984; Dikötter 2017). Qingyi's parents were under great strain and refused to talk to their children about what was happening around them. She and her siblings soon learned to stop asking questions. Classes ceased at both the vocational and primary school at some point in the late 1960s—Qingyi does not remember exactly when—and the children's days were filled with unsupervised play, with long hours spent wandering around the school campus and surrounding neighborhoods by themselves.

In 1974, Qingyi left her family to live and work in a farming village. She did not go willingly; she was compelled by Mao Zedong's rustication movement, in which millions of urban youths were "sent down" to the countryside in order to be "educated" by the peasantry (see Honig and Zhao 2015). She was just seventeen years old when she left her family behind. Qingyi was fortunate in that her assigned village was close enough to Chengdu that she could visit home once a month or so. Her brothers were sent to villages so far away that she only saw them once a year. Qingyi told me that this wasn't a coincidence. Her parents were able to pull some strings to keep one of their children nearby. They chose her because she was a girl, and they worried she wouldn't acclimate to the countryside as well as her brothers.

Working alongside farmers was indeed mentally and physically grueling. Qingyi recalls toiling for 10–12 hours in the fields by day and sleeping in a poorly constructed mud house with three other "sent down" youths by night. All of them were young women from urban families, and none had been properly taught how to cook, much less build a fire in the house's wood-fired stove. They ate nothing but burned rice and boiled greens for dinner every evening for the first few months. Winter months were frigid, and the roof often leaked. When the weather warmed, their straw beds jumped with fleas. Four years of Qingyi's life were spent like this.

The winds of change finally began to blow in 1978, two years after Mao's death and with the ascension of his reform-minded successor Deng Xiaoping. Though Qingyi had never enjoyed studying, she was glad when her parents called in some favors to secure a seat for her at a vocational school in Chengdu. She was among the fortunate: many sent-down youths never got the chance to go home. Qingyi began a course in accounting at the vocation school, and then met a man who would later become her husband. After graduating in 1980, she was assigned to a work unit at a state-owned enterprise (SOE) that designed and produced large farm machinery. Her husband, who trained in engineering, was assigned to the same factory in a different department. Qingyi had no particular desire to be an accountant and had no interest in farm equipment. None of these personal preferences mattered. The Chinese work-unit system was developed to achieve full urban employment and guaranteed employment for life; the trade-off was that people had very little choice in the type of employment they received.

Qingyi told me she bore all of these major life changes reasonably well. She had a strong constitution and seemed to adjust to each transition without much fuss. "Some of the other girls," she said, "they would cry in the dormitories at the school and then in the factory because they missed home or because they had a fight with somebody. But I never let those things bother me." When Qingyi and her husband married in 1981, they moved out of the factory dormitories and into her husband's parents' apartment. The first time that her confidence was seriously shaken was in 1982, when she became seriously ill from a high-risk pregnancy that ended in a dangerous labor and delivery. "Everyone thought I was going to die," she recalled. However, she was young, healthy, and recovered more quickly than anyone expected. She returned to work at the factory within months. It would be her only pregnancy: because all of her reproductive years coincided with the one-child policy, Qingyi and her husband are among the millions of urban Chinese couples who have a single child.

Qingyi described being forced to retire as the second time that her confidence was tested, and she attributed her inability to shake off the transition to her age: "You're weaker when you get older," she said. "Maybe if I had been younger I wouldn't have taken it so hard." When I first met Qingyi in 2014, she had already been out of work for about fifteen years. In 1999, when she was just forty-two years old, her factory was swept up in the wave of economic reforms that was then transforming cities throughout the country. In its bid to modernize the Chinese economy, the state privatized, shuttered, or restructured thousands of state-owned enterprises (Chiu and Hung 2004; Song 2003). Qingyi's factory downsized and moved from an industrial area in eastern Chengdu to a new industrial zone south of the city; while her husband kept his job, she, along with hundreds of other employees, was sent home with a meager 10,000 RMB (about 1,200 USD in 1999) severance pay. Having grown up in her father's work unit, then packed off to the countryside as a sent-down youth, then assigned to a job in a state-owned factory upon finishing vocational school, Qingyi had never known a life outside of state control. Her life, up until that point, was like a conveyor belt that transported her from one stage to the next without her input.

Being unemployed was a serious blow not only to Qingyi's self-confidence but also to her sense of personal identity. She had thought she would have that job until she died, or at least until she became incapacitated by illness or old age. Instead, at the prime of her life, social forces beyond her control prevented Qingyi from contributing to her family's financial security. More significantly, they stripped her of a defined social role. "I avoided meeting new people during those years," Qingyi recalled. "People would ask about what I did, and I would feel so stupid because I wouldn't know what to say. You can't say you're a retiree when you're in your forties." Pushed out of the workforce in a society that increasingly used economic productivity as a key indicator of success, Qingyi felt like her life had been marginalized and devalued. At the same time, due to her relatively young age, she did not feel at ease taking on a "retiree" identity. Like many other urbanites, Qingyi had taken the Chinese Communist Party's promise that residents would be taken care of "from the cradle to the grave" at face value (Leung 1994; Ma 2006). When this promise was broken, Qingyi was sent adrift, with little idea of what to do with her remaining years.

Looking at her now, one would have a hard time imagining what Qingyi was like in those listless years. Her commanding presence fills any room she enters: she dresses in bright, colorful clothing and speaks with effusive energy. Her social life revolves almost exclusively around her dance group, and she can frequently be found in the company of women like herself. In other words, Qingyi is a typical *dama*—the colloquial term in China for women in late middle age who spend their time enjoying themselves in congregational dance groups.

Facing Choices in Mid-life

Because so many others were similarly impacted by the same wide-reaching policies, Qingyi's life history offers an incisive view into the experiences of women of her generation. As a cohort, they have endured some of the most significant changes of China's recent history during their lifetimes. Though the details varied—the name of the village to which they were "sent down," the name of the factory where they were assigned a job, the year of their marriage—I was struck again and again by the overwhelming similarities among my interlocutors' accounts of their lives leading up to their premature exits from the work force. An estimated seventy-two million people lost their jobs due to SOE reforms between the late 1990s and early 2000s (Whyte 2012). The layoffs not only caused high unemployment rates in urban areas but also disproportionately affected female workers, who tended to hold lower-skill, lower-wage positions (Du and Dong 2009; Kong, Osberg, and Zhou 2019). This means that at the turn of the millennium, there were millions of able-bodied middle-aged people—most of them women—living in Chinese cities with very little to do.

For Qingyi and millions of other women, broad social changes and economic reforms dislocated them from the life trajectory they thought they were on and left them to figure out the rest on their own. Scholarly conversations about China's social transformations tend to focus on the practical consequences of Deng Xiaoping's economic policy reforms. Policy changes that culminated in the smashing of the so-called iron rice bowl in urban areas included radical measures to privatize health care, education, and housing (see Tang and Parish 2000). Most urbanites experienced the effects of these reforms in multiple dimensions of their lives: public housing was replaced with a booming real estate market; urban workers were either laid off or were no longer guaranteed jobs and benefits for life; family structures altered as young couples began to prefer homes of their own to traditional multigenerational households. Taken together, these changes amounted to a comprehensive restructuring of the public domain.

However, there are other dimensions of post-reform life in China that deserve further scrutiny—namely, ordinary people's efforts to make sense of their surroundings and remake themselves for this new reality. Despite a major reordering of state-society relations, China never underwent a regime change. Today, the People's Republic of China remains a socialist state. The technical term for China's current form of governance is "socialism with Chinese characteristics," which is meant to describe the current mixed economy that features a strong central government directing the forces of the market. This does not mean, however, that people who lived through China's economic reforms experienced a sense of continuity. In public culture, the psychological ramifications of undergoing rapid ideological transition have been explored widely in multiple genres in China since the beginning of the so-called ideological "thaw" that began with Mao's death in 1976. Though well-known artistic movements that sprung up during this period (such as "scar literature" and "fifth-generation" filmmaking) did not necessarily take overtly critical stances toward socialism, the new generation of writers and artists often created plot lines without clear-cut heroes or villains and instead focused on the suffering of ordinary people. In doing so, they created art that lacked the ideological purity of its collective-era predecessors, which invariably pitted "good" forces (peasants, the Communist Party) against "evil" ones (landlords, capitalists, the Nationalist Party, and the Japanese).

It is difficult to gauge the impacts of representational media on the average person's psyche, but reform policies' repercussions for private lives also manifested in clearly observable ways. Sociologist Fei Xiaotong noted in the 1930s that Chinese society is organized on a set of differential social hierarchies with the individual at the center. The centrality of the individual in this model means something quite counterintuitive to the Western observer: the circles denote levels of obligation a person has toward their relations (Fei 1992). These hierarchies' power in mediating social relations cannot be overstated: under this system, all acquaintances were addressed by a kinship term according to his or her age and station, and afforded the respect (or lack thereof) commensurate with that station. This family system has not existed in its pure form (if such a thing ever existed) for quite some time: it was first replaced by communist ideologies of kinship based on Marxist-Leninist principles, which made all citizens members of a communist "brotherhood" with the state acting as the all-knowing father figure at its head. Economic reforms—as well as the one-child policy—introduced new and complex changes. The nuclear family became more important, young people gained more social power, and the emotional aspects of relationships became more and more emphasized (Fong 2004; Santos and Harrell Santos 2016; Kuan 2015).

These so-called modern social processes did not supplant traditional ones overnight. In his work on social change in rural China, Yunxiang Yan (2003) notes that a few customs, such as intergenerational households living together in large one-room family homes, did disappear altogether. However, most traditional practices like dowry transfers and certain wedding rituals either persisted in modified form or were given new social meanings. In another study on rural China, Xin Liu (2000) similarly observed that the transition between the collective and reform eras was by no means linear. There was, instead, a loosening-up of cultural expectations around relationships and rituals, and people were often left to their own devices to weave a coherent social fabric together from a jumbled assortment of behaviors and practices. In other words, there was never a clean break between "traditional" social frameworks and "modern" ones; it would be more accurate to say that a single way of life was replaced with multiple competing and at times contradictory choices.

When I asked retirees about what it was like to live through the early decades of economic reforms, almost every interviewee mentioned the rapid expansion of new choices in some capacity. Most people spoke in reference to the new consumer and cultural goods—clothes, food, music, cars, housing, hairstyles, furniture, the list goes on—that became available when Deng Xiaoping reopened China to foreign business and influence. I also have my own memories of this time. I was five or six years old when the first Western-style supermarket opened in Chengdu in the early 1990s. My mother took me there one day after school as a special treat. The store was very small by today's standards, but it was novel in that all the products were displayed in open aisles rather than behind counters. My mother told me I could choose one thing to buy. Upon surveying the vast options of chips, candy, and other snacks on display, some of which I had never seen before, I became overwhelmed by indecision and burst into tears.

Of course, this rather pitiful childhood experience captures only a slim shadow of what Deborah Davis (2000) has dubbed China's "consumer revolution." The reality is that economic reforms transformed the very fabric of daily life. In her work on the rise of the real estate market in urban China, Li Zhang (2010) astutely notes that the work-unit or *danwei* system did not simply provide jobs and housing to urban workers, but was rather a comprehensive mechanism of social organization that limited personal choices and brought the bulk of daily affairs (like health care, recreation, and childcare) under state control (also see Walder 1983; Bray 2005; Cliff 2015). When the *danwei* system began to wane and as people increasingly moved into privately purchased homes, they also began to gain personal autonomy in many of these affairs for the first time (see Derleth and Koldyk 2004). All this is to say that in addition to having higher salaries and greater access to consumer goods, consumption has become, as Lisa Rofel (2007) puts it, a vehicle for "embodying a new self" in post-reform society (118).

For people like Qingyi, all of this was occurring just as they were entering mid-life, and moreover just as they became untethered from the job—and therefore social institution—they thought they could rely on for life. How does one go about embodying a new self under these circumstances? How does one do it without crying from the sheer exhaustion of having to make so many new choices?

Choosing to Play, Choosing to Dance

When Qingyi's generation was young, life oftentimes felt oppressive and at times even brutal. However, it offered a sort of all-encompassing clarity that can no longer be found in any area of post-reform society. When I asked what she had wanted to be if not an accountant, Qingyi shrugged. "I never thought about it," she said. "We didn't think about this kind of thing when we were young." Since they had so few opportunities to cultivate their own interests or choose their own paths in life, many simply did not bother. When they were laid off from their jobs, however, they were left with no choice but to think about what they actually wanted to do with their lives. Some, out of necessity or desire, got new jobs. Private enterprises were booming in the aftermath of economic reforms, and finding new employment was definitely possible for those who had marketable skills or were able to retrain. A few women I spoke to even took advantage of the entrepreneurial atmosphere and started their own businesses during this period. Some others were content to stay home and live a quieter life taking care of family members. Many of them, however, decided they wanted to dance.

I cannot pinpoint the definitive year or date for the origin of the congregational dancing phenomenon because it did not develop overnight. Group public exercise has been a common sight in China since at least the early twentieth century, when Republican nation-building efforts began to emphasize physical prowess as a means to establish China's dominance on the global stage (Morris 2004). The development of a politically inflected physical culture continued under the CCP, when people regularly performed Soviet-style group calisthenics with other members of their work units or schools (Brownell 1995; Shen and Fan 2021). The Cultural Revolution era saw the rise of revolutionary ballet. Troupes of Red Guards—teenage devotees of Mao Zedong and his teachings—would perform works like "The Red Detachment of Women" to official audiences as well as on the streets. Then, in the earlier years of the reform era, there was a resurgence of interest in traditional mind-body exercises like tai chi and qigong. The latter became so popular in the 1980s and 1990s that David Palmer (2007) dubbed it a "qigong fever" that only subsided when certain groups—chief among them the Falun Gong sect, became politically suspect.

The congregational dancing phenomenon has features in common with each of these previous forms of public exercise. In fact, many Chinese internet commentators and younger people I spoke to subscribed to the belief that congregational dancers were revolutionary ballet performers in their youth and simply continued the habit after retirement. There is little evidence to support this theory: there are far more congregational dancers than there were Red Guards, and it's quite obvious that most people who participate in congregational dance groups have no former dance training. Despite the fact that the phenomenon has no clear starting point, most people seem to agree that dance groups made up of middle-aged women became ubiquitous at some point in the early 2000s. At first, the groups tended to consist of 10–20 people who danced together in public parks. Of the groups I surveyed during my preliminary research, a vast majority—over 80 percent—began as a gathering of a small group of women who were laid off from the same companies. These types of groups gradually expanded as founding members brought in friends or neighbors who were also newly unemployed. Even more people joined as women who reached official retirement age—as young as fifty—joined the ranks of those who were laid off prematurely.

Over the years, the phenomenon grew to be so massive that it transformed the sensory experience of living in a Chinese city. Between 7 A.M. and 9 A.M., and again between 6 P.M. and 9 P.M., nearly all of Chengdu's public parks and riverbank esplanade fill with the sights and sounds of people dancing. The more popular spots where multiple groups gather right next to each other produce a cacophony of discordant beats. Many dancers like to wear bright colors and provide a colorful visual spectacle as they move in sync. Some groups show up for their practices donning matching outfits. A black jersey top paired with a pink-and-red floral skirt is one popular getup; stretch knit matching sets with a single accent color along the collar and down the leg of the pants were also commonly seen. There are shops and online markets that cater exclusively to congregational dancers, and these retailers all seemed to sell the same wares, so many dance groups end up looking identical to one another. Depending on the type of dance they are doing, some groups also carry props like handheld fans, silk scarves, umbrellas, or even tennis rackets as part of their routines.

Because the phenomenon consists of a hundred million participants scattered across the most populous country in the world, it is also incredibly diverse. Groups of 10–30 women are still common, though there is so much variation that I hesitate to call them "typical." Some groups consist of just three or four members, while others are so large that they can fill expansive city squares. Some blast their music loudly and seem to relish the attention they receive from passersby, while others prefer secluded spaces away from the public eye. Groups can also differ wildly in terms of dance style. A large number—perhaps a small majority—favor traditional Chinese dance. This is a loaded term that means different things to different people, but I use it to refer to a collection of styles based on folk dance that have been subsumed into official definitions of "Chinese dance" by state-sponsored dance institutions (Wilcox 2018b). Ballroom and Latin dance styles are also quite popular; men who participate in congregational dancing tend to gravitate toward these groups since male dance partners are highly coveted. Finally, there is a wide range in degree of physical intensity of movements. On one end of the spectrum, there are groups for whom aerobic exercise, rather than aesthetic enjoyment, is the primary objective. Their movements resemble those that might be found in a Western cardio-dance or Zumba class and are sometimes performed with light dumbbells. On the other end of the spectrum, some groups simply gather to walk a few rhythmic steps in place while chatting with each other. All these distinctions motivated me to call the phenomenon "congregational dancing" rather than "public dancing" or "square dancing"; the only true overlap I can identify between all groups is that they bring people together.

By the time I began my research, the phenomenon had fully integrated into the daily rhythm of the city, acting like semipermanent fixtures of the urban landscape. I stayed in an apartment on the thirty-third floor of an apartment building during my fieldwork, and the sound of music blasting from a dance group's portable speaker was often the first thing I heard in the morning. The groups also made use of commercial areas, parking lots, and sidewalks. On my twice-weekly excursion to the local market to buy groceries—a walk that took eight minutes—I would pass the same twelve dance groups again and again. Sometimes, after visiting my grandmother on the other side of the city or a dinner out with a friend, I would elect to walk home along the riverside esplanade rather than take the bus. I learned to mark distances by the appearances of certain groups: seeing the salsa dancers bedecked in glittering skirts meant that I was halfway there, and I was just ten minutes from home when I reached the women wearing matching sweatbands with the particularly loud pop music.

I knew it would not be possible to get an in-depth look at every kind of congregational dance group during the duration of my fieldwork, but I still tried to select groups with different organizing structures and priorities. I ended up joining two groups for most of a year: the "Dancing Beauties" and the "Sunset Dance Group." The latter group consisted of about twenty women in their mid- to late sixties. They were a neighborhood group, meaning that all the women lived within walking distance to the park where their daily dances were held. The women in the Dancing Beauties were a few years younger, with a median age of sixty-one. They were also wealthier, on account of having held higher-paying jobs prior to retirement. This relative privilege allowed them to be more discerning in their choice of meeting venue: they danced weekly in a private indoors dance studio expressly to avoid the noise and regulations of public spaces.

The Dancing Beauties rented a shared studio space and had exclusive use of one of three large and airy studios on the third floor of a four-story building from 4:20 P.M. until 6:20 P.M. on every Thursday afternoon. The three nearly identical studios have windows overlooking a tree-lined riverbank and full-length mirrors lining one of the walls and ballet barres lining the three others. Besides the Dancing Beauties, Thursday afternoons on the third floor also hosted a yoga class (attended exclusively by young women) as well as two children's ballet classes. The building was a bustling place. Though we never crossed paths with them, the studio manager told me that two other groups of *dama*—the colloquial term for retired women who participate in congregational dancing—also held classes in the same studio on different days of the week. People changing shoes and clothes crowded the narrow hallways before and after each class; young girls in tutus often snuck into the studio at 6:15 and giggled until the Dancing Beauties yielded the space to them.

Despite the chaos, the Dancing Beauties counted themselves lucky to have found the space: it was the third dance studio that the group had occupied since its members started dancing together in 2011. They lost one space because the rent had doubled, and another because the building that housed it was slated for demolition. This studio was close to public transit, well-maintained, and at 100 RMB per hour, quite affordable. Every ten weeks, the Dancing Beauties' group leader, a woman in her mid-sixties whom everyone called Teacher Yuan, collected 120 RMB from each group member to pay for ten sessions in advance. There was invariably money left over, and Teacher Yuan reserved these excess funds to pay for group outings, meals, and parties. Even though she collected dues and ran the classes, Teacher Yuan never kept any money for herself or took payment for her work. She once explained to me that this was because she wanted the Dancing Beauties to feel like a friend group rather than a formal class: "If I took money like a regular dance teacher, then the whole feeling of the group would change. I prefer it this way."

There was no uniform, but everyone came each week wearing very similar clothes: exercise pants and leather-soled dance slippers with T-shirts in the summer and wool sweaters in the winter. People also made sure to bring dance props like umbrellas, fans, and silk scarves.

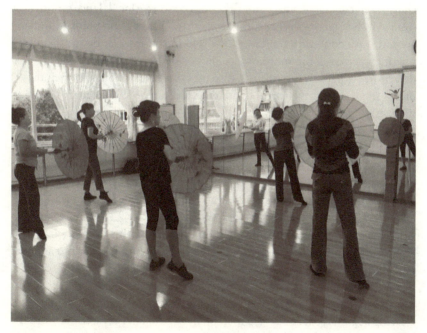

FIGURE 2 Members of the Dancing Beauties practicing in their rented studio space. (Photo by Claudia Huang)

The Dancing Beauties practiced traditional Chinese dance. The two-hour-long classes always began with form drills, with everyone standing in the first balletic position (feet pointing outward, back straight, tail tucked) with hands on the barre and facing the mirrored walls. After turning on the music on her portable speaker set, Teacher Yuan walked around the room inspecting our postures and issued various commands: "Stand up straighter!" "You—shoulders back!" "You must make more of an effort to bring your knees together!" When she was satisfied that we were all in the best first positions that we could muster, we would continue to other movements. For about an hour, we performed barre exercises like pliés and arabesques that aimed to stretch, warm, and tone our muscles on Teacher Yuan's cues. Though I was the youngest person in the class by several decades, Teacher Yuan's dance drills were no walk in the park for me. I often struggled through the grueling leg extensions and would leave class drenched in sweat during the summer.

For the first three months that I was in the class, Teacher Yuan seemed to single me out for gentle yet persistent criticism. "You must lift your chest and keep your tail down. You must control your mid-section. Only then will the flavor come out." This flavor, this *weidao,* was one of Teacher Yuan's favorite refrains. She frequently invoked it when extolling the virtues of taking a dance class that focuses on mastering foundational ballet movements, especially when compared with run-of-the-mill congregational dance groups that (in her mind) ignore bodily form altogether. "There is no point in moving around if it's done with no flavor," she told me on my first day as she disapprovingly assessed my movements. She assured me, however, that natural defects in my posture (too casual), hips (not controlled enough in their movement), and shoulders (too muscular) could all be corrected by dancing diligently.

Every woman in the group took the classes seriously. A few of them had danced a bit when they were younger, but none had been formally trained. Nevertheless, the group made an earnest effort each week to improve. People encouraged and critiqued each other's movements. Though the room buzzed with gossip and chatter before class began and after it ended, everyone was quiet and attentive whenever Teacher Yuan spoke.

By contrast, the Sunset Dance Group operated with a far more informal atmosphere. They danced every morning in a little park tucked into an older neighborhood with crowded narrow streets. The park itself was humble: it boasted some rusty exercise equipment, a few wooden benches, and a tiled clearing approximately the size of a basketball court. The group danced in this clearing beginning at about 8:30 A.M. each day, though they were far from the only people using the park at that time. On any given morning, groups of small children ran about playing on the exercise equipment, couples sat on the wooden benches sipping on tea from their thermoses, and shoppers used the dance space as a shortcut from the street to an open-air produce market that stood directly adjacent to the park.

The proximity of the dance space to the market was both a blessing and a curse. On the one hand, the space was always chaotic, and at least once per morning the group would be interrupted by a gaggle of running children, absent-minded shoppers too busy scrolling their phones to notice their surroundings, or a street merchant with a loudspeaker affixed to his bicycle handlebars blasting out advertisements for his wares at full volume. On the other hand, most members of the Sunset Dance Group, myself included, made good use of the market by going shopping for fresh produce every day. This was a habit I picked up from the group: while most people my age in Chengdu did their shopping in the big international supermarkets that had sprung up everywhere in recent years, older residents often retained the custom of shopping for ingredients each morning in open-air neighborhood markets. By going dancing each morning, we also got our meal planning out of the way.

The exposed and public nature of the group's meeting space has other implications for how the group operates. The small park also serves as a community-gathering place during holidays and special events. Over the years, the Sunset Dance Group has been repeatedly called upon to perform at these events and, in the course of their interactions with local officials about the events, have also been recruited to compete in local congregational dancing competitions. By 2017, the group's daily practices practically revolved around preparing for either competitions or community performances, and the local community (*shequ*) government was so involved with the group's goings-on that four *shequ* officials were permanent members of the Sunset Dance Groups' WeChat messaging group.

Like the Dancing Beauties, the Sunset Dance Group favored traditional Chinese dances (though it also dabbled in other genres on occasion). Unlike the Dancing Beauties, the Sunset Dance group did not have a regular teacher who was present for all meetings. Instead, it hired a semiprofessional dancer named Teacher Wang to teach them a new dance on the first Wednesday of each month, paying her a small fee for her time. On all other days, group members collectively decided what they wanted to practice, usually choosing a mix of pieces that the women were still learning as well as pieces that the entire group was already familiar with. More competent dancers stood at the front of the group so that others could emulate them, while beginners—like myself—and less dexterous dancers stood at the back so as to not confuse others with their movements. In general, however, people in the Sunset Dance Group were not concerned with posture or positioning: everyone simply showed up each day to try her best, and no one was chastised for subpar dancing. There was no official end time to the daily meetings, but the women generally began to disband at around 10 A.M. to allow ample time to shop and prepare lunch.

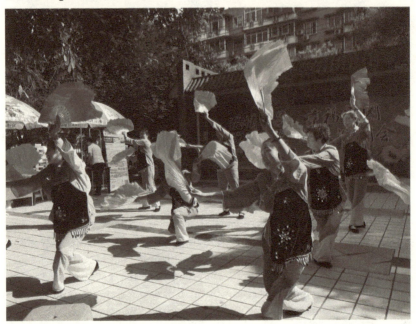

FIGURE 3 Members of the Sunset Dance Group performing at a community holiday event. (Photo by Claudia Huang)

Despite these differences between the two groups, the women who belonged to them had a lot in common with each other. They were all middle-aged or a little older: in 2017, the oldest was seventy-two years old and the was youngest fifty-six years old. They were all retired or had been laid off during SOE reforms (though a few had found new jobs afterward). Except for the seventy-two-year-old, who had her children before the one-child policy was enacted, and another woman who spent her childbearing years in a rural village where the policy was not strictly enforced, they all had just one child. Their parents were in their eighties and nineties and were rapidly declining in both health and the ability to live independently. They all invested a lot of emotional energy into their dance groups and organized their social lives around the other women in their groups. They all loved congregational dancing, even if they did not particularly enjoy all the different pieces that go into it.

In case it is not already clear, I really enjoyed spending time with the congregational dancers. Chengdu has always been a dynamic place, but the dancers made the city feel more alive, more fun. Not everyone shares my enthusiasm. Since the early 2000s but especially starting in the mid-2010s, there have been regular media (and, later, social media) reports of clashes between dance groups and urban dwellers who cannot stand their noise. Such reports tend to highlight the most sensational conflicts, like the time irritated residents in

Changsha pelted dancers with human feces (Carter 2013), or the time a man in Guangxi opened fire on a group and shot a dancer in the leg (Buckley 2016). In my own observations, however, tensions manifest much more frequently in the form of kvetching among groups of friends or posting complaints online in search of sympathy. Many people I spoke to in Chengdu sympathized with the fact that retirees needed something to do but at the same time resented them for taking up so much space and disturbing the peace with their noise. In keeping with the popular notion that congregational dancers were former Red Guards, or at least enthusiastic participants in the political turmoil of the Cultural Revolution, these complaints often contained the same refrain: "It's not that old people became bad, it's that bad people became old."

While I do not agree with their sentiments, I can see why detractors are upset. I also did not appreciate being woken up by loud music every morning. I am sure I would have been even more annoyed if I had been trying to sleep off a night shift or calm a fussy infant. Dance groups can also be quite disruptive to day-to-day activities. For example, I lived near a shopping center that abutted a large paved plaza. During the day, the plaza was mostly empty save for people playing fetch with their dogs or office workers stopping momentarily to eat lunch on one of the benches scattered about. But in the evenings, a group of about 200 women in matching yellow T-shirts took over this space to do jazz-inspired cardio-step dance exercises. Anyone wanting to go into the shopping center needed to weave through this rhythmic crowd, taking special care to not get smacked in the face by someone's jazz hands. I found it difficult enough as a young, able-bodied person, and imagine that it would have been quite impossible if I had any kind of mobility issue or cared for someone who did.

For these reasons, congregational dancers are frequently accused of being selfish (Huang 2016). While no congregational dancer I met would accept such a characterization, it is certainly true that many of them cherish their newfound ability to try out and cultivate personal identities based on their own interests and tastes. Sometimes, when speaking with someone complaining about dance groups, I would attempt to explain this angle to them. On more than one occasion, my interlocutor would then demand to know why retired women could not choose more private and less noisy activities. The truth is that many of them do.

Take, for example, a woman I call Auntie Zhang. Her story is a familiar one: having worked at a state-owned company her entire adult life, she was laid off along with hundreds of her colleagues in 2003 when she was forty-four years old. In the years following the layoff, she became so bored and aimless that, in her own words, she started to feel like she was losing her mind. When the situation became untenable, she decided that she was going to spend time learning things that she did not have the time or resources to learn when she was young. She enrolled at a local "old age university"—an institution of learning specially devoted to retirees—as soon as she qualified and signed up for as many classes as she was allowed to take. Soon, her days were full.

In the fall 2016, Auntie Zhang invited me to join her at the university's thirtieth-anniversary exhibition. The event was held in a large auditorium and an adjoining gallery space on the university's campus. The latter showcased students' paintings, drawings, calligraphy, and digital artwork, while live performances were held in the former. As we sat together in the back row of the jam-packed auditorium, Auntie Zhang told me that she was taking four different classes per week: two dance classes (one Latin, one ballet), photography on Thursday mornings, and calligraphy on Tuesday afternoons. On Saturdays, she went on to explain, she walked in the countryside with a walking group formed from among her classmates at the university. "And so now the only days that are empty are Wednesdays and Sundays," she said. "All in all," she finished smiling, "I feel quite busy!"

The Chengdu Old Age University is just one of three learning centers reserved for older adults and retirees, and there are an estimated seventy thousand such institutions throughout China. Like all other institutions of its type, the Chengdu Old Age University has one major problem: overcrowding. Class fees are quite affordable, and people only need to meet the official retirement age to enroll. Because China's population is rapidly aging, and because retirement ages are set so low, more people qualify every year. In an interview, the vice principal of the Chengdu university smiled wanly as she told me a joke that she had undoubtedly told dozens if not hundreds of times before: "We get new students every year, but no one ever graduates." People routinely line up outside the school gates at midnight on the first day of the enrollment period to get their first picks of classes. The most popular classes, such as piano and tai chi, the vice principal explained, have hundreds of people on their waiting lists. To serve more students, the university instituted new rules in 2017 that limit each person to two courses per semester and kicks people out after they have completed a three-course series on the same subject. But the lines persist, and there are never enough classes to go around. There simply is not enough supply to meet the demand of so many retirees seeking fulfillment and community.

Congregational dance groups offer something old age universities, community centers, and other programming aimed at older adults cannot: near-universal accessibility and customizability. There are groups in virtually every corner of the city, and there are so many different types that most people can find one that suits them provided they are willing to move their bodies a little. Though almost all groups charge fees to pay for shared expenses like props and speakers, the amount is usually quite small—on average a few hundred RMB per year—and it is not necessary to stand in line to gain entry. They also offer the sort of consistency that many older adults miss after leaving the workforce.

Groups meet at the same time each day or week, and members see familiar faces on a regular basis.

That said, people join dance groups for many different reasons. I received a wide variety of replies when I surveyed people about their motivations for dancing as part of my preliminary research. Many mentioned wanting to exercise, but their reasons for exercising also varied: some were trying to lose weight, some wanted to remain healthy in order to not be a burden on their children, and some wanted to manage chronic conditions like hypertension or high cholesterol. A significant portion of respondents said that they joined to alleviate post-retirement boredom. A few were quite blunt about the instrumental role that their group played in their lives: when I was interviewing Auntie Deng, for example, another woman stood nearby and chimed in when she heard Auntie Deng talking about her daily routine. This woman was a widow and lived alone. She explained in a half-joking manner that she joined the dance group so that if she collapsed in her apartment one day, her absence would be noticed. These responses were not mutually exclusive, of course, and most people reported having more than one motivation.

For all the women in both the Sunset Dance Group and the Dancing Beauties, joining a congregational dancing group opened their lives to new experiences, friendships, and pursuits of meaning. As I have previously noted, congregational dance groups act as both social anchors and social launchpads. Members frequently get together for meals and other social activities, creating a sense of stable community. Perhaps more importantly, they also offer each other support and encouragement to pursue personal interests, whatever those might be (Huang 2016). Most women in both groups took classes at various old age universities or community centers. (In fact, I unexpectedly ran into a member of the Dancing Beauties at the exhibition I attended with Auntie Zhang. She was there to showcase some of her work from her fashion design class.) In the case of both groups, a few women began taking classes first, and the rest soon followed after hearing favorable reports. Through the connections they made in their groups, many also became members of other social collectives like choirs, bird-watching meetups, and karaoke clubs. The congregational dancing phenomenon pushed a critical mass of retirees with similar life experiences together, which in turn created opportunities for new alliances to form. During my preliminary research period, for example, I briefly spent time with a dining club made up of women from three different dance groups that used the same park. They called themselves the "half off sisters" because they only ate at restaurants that offered senior citizens a 50 percent discount. In another instance, three members of a dance group bonded over their shared Buddhist faith and began accompanying each other to lectures and temple events. These other less-visible interests do not garner nearly as much attention as congregational dancing, but they are very much part of the same story of retired Chinese women's pursuit of midlife revival.

Interestingly, while almost everyone I surveyed referred to the aesthetic dimensions of congregational dancing in some way—that they found the music enjoyable, that they liked wearing the costumes or uniforms, that they liked learning to move in a different way—no one said they joined a dance group because they liked dancing per se. Instead, as Auntie Deng put it, congregational dance groups offer their participants a sense of purpose—whatever that may mean to individual people. The congregational dancing phenomenon did not grow to be so massive because an entire generation of people somehow came to prefer dancing above all other pastimes. Instead, its origins lie in the social and historical circumstances that left this generation unmoored. Without the need to adhere to strict narratives about how life should unfold, people are now free to imagine a wide variety of possible futures and forms of happiness and meaning. Though there are no guarantees of success, they can now at least try to cultivate themselves, and their lives, on their own terms.

2

Dama Mania

• • • • • • • • • • • • • • • • • • • •

Chengdu has a subtropical climate with cool, mild winters and oppressively hot summers. On the hottest days, when the air hangs so thick that not even the cicadas seem to move, all but the most dedicated dance groups are forced to cancel practice. On such a day in July 2016, I got word from the Sunset Dance Group that practice was canceled when I was already on the bus headed toward the park. Not wanting to waste the day, I decided to visit my grandmother instead. I disembarked from my bus and boarded another one headed toward my grandmother's neighborhood, only to find that a small group of older men had commandeered all the seats in the back. Judging by their casual sleeveless shirts, tea thermoses, plastic bags of sunflower seeds, and bamboo hand-held fans, they were likely headed to a park or teahouse to while the day away. The bus was not crowded, but the men filled the space with raucous noise as they sat joking and boasting with their belongings scattered about the seats around them. In both appearance and manner, they fulfilled nearly every local stereotype about a certain class of retired men: brash, uncouth, and connoisseurs of leisure. They briefly paused their conversation at each stop to gaze at the people coming aboard to ascertain whether they needed to yield any seats, and then resumed talking when the bus drove on. At one stop, a woman wearing a stylish summer dress with oversized sunglasses embarked. Her hair was permed, braided, and coifed into an elaborate design at the nape of her neck. She looked to be about forty-five. However, when she swiped her bus pass on the electronic payment kiosk, the machine's automated female voice announced "*laonian ka*," or Senior Card.

As is the case in many cities across China, older adults in Chengdu over the age of seventy are entitled to ride public transportation for free with a so-called Senior Card transit pass (though in some cities the age to be considered "senior" is sixty-five). It is a benefit provided by the municipal government to reduce the cost of living for retirees and encourage them to remain active in their communities. For the men sitting in the back of the bus, however, the card offered another, more subtle benefit—a public clue about the age of their fellow bus passengers. "She's old like us!" I heard one of them say to the others as we rolled away from the stop, "but you would have never known had it not been for her bus pass. She looks like she's going to her office job!" At this, all the men in the group roared in laughter. "We have to be thankful for the bus passes," another man added. "People are so well-preserved now. You can't tell just by looking anymore." They each nodded and chuckled in agreement before moving on to another topic. The woman in question, who was talking on the phone at the front of the bus, was too far away to take note of the commotion her entrance had momentarily caused, but for me, witnessing this episode opened many questions about how old age is understood, demarcated, and treated in China today. If the external markers of old age are no longer agreed upon or stable, then how do people know when they have become old? How did this destabilization of age-graded categories come to be, and what confusions or anxieties are produced as a result? Finally, what new ways of being old are created amid this confusion?

This chapter provides some answers to these questions by examining the *dama* stereotype that is so closely associated with the congregational dancing phenomenon. Typically, a *dama* is a woman in her fifties, sixties, or early seventies. In China, people of this age are considered to be *zhong laonian,* or "older middle-aged," but not everyone in the age cohort is a *dama*. Shortly before leaving Chengdu at the end of 2017, I sent an informal survey to some friends on the popular Chinese messaging platform WeChat. This survey contained only one question: "How would you describe a *dama*?" The answers returned almost immediately: "A late–middle-aged woman who likes to pose for photos in bright scarves." "Someone who likes to dance with other old ladies." "Women who talk loudly with drawn-on eyebrows." "My mother." I queried a wide variety of acquaintances—colleagues from Sichuan University, my cousins, shop owners I'd come to know, older relatives, and expats—not because I did not understand the term but because I wanted to assess the recognizability of the *dama* stereotype. The differences in people's responses did not catch my attention as much as the fact that nearly everyone who received the question offered an answer. The specifics varied, but each person held a clear and developed picture of a *dama* in his or her mind's eye. On another occasion, my friend Xia—an educated and well-traveled woman in her late twenties, told me that it is impossible to pin down an exact description of *dama* because "they like to dress differently for different occasions," but that "you know one when you see one."

As is often the case when people are recognized and marked by shared pastimes, aesthetic preferences, and social circles, the *dama* stereotype reveals less about the people belonging to the category and more about implicit or unspoken systems of values that govern the society from which the stereotype emerged (see Quillian and Pager 2001). Even though the term *dama* has only been in wide circulation for about a decade, it has already made an indelible mark on the popular imagination. *Dama* [大妈] literally translates to "big mother" but means something closer to "auntie." References to *dama* make regular appearances in magazines, blogs, online commentaries, and even state-sponsored variety shows, often in the form of jokes poking fun at the women's clothing or mannerisms. Among Chinese urbanites and on the Chinese web, *dama* has become a shorthand for a certain type of woman—retired, late–middle-aged or a little older, colorfully attired and colorfully outspoken, and often in the company of women like herself. She is urban but not urbane. She favors bright scarves and permed hair. She enjoys shopping, but never buys anything at full price. She does not mind attracting the attention of strangers.

Despite the humor and even silliness of many of these discussions, I believe they point to the emergence of a serious and far-reaching social discourse on what it means to grow old—particularly as a woman—in the People's Republic of China today. Calling an older woman a *dama* is seldom a compliment. By favoring fashions and grooming practices usually considered more appropriate for younger women and by continuing to participate in public life, women identified as *dama* do not fit the traditional mold of the dignified, family-oriented aging matriarch. At the same time, because they tend to live on fixed incomes and are perceived to cling to collective activities that harken back to the Mao era, women identified as *dama* also fail to achieve the model of self-sufficient "successful" aging that became prominent in the aftermath of China's economic reforms (Chen and Chen 2009; Powell 2012). My goal here is not to tame the mercurial nature of the *dama* stereotype or to mine the wide range of personal impressions for patterns in hopes of giving it a definite shape. Instead, I use the stereotype to argue that a newly recognized category of older woman has emerged in Chinese society today, and that this emergence points to deeper social changes.

My reasons for doing so are twofold: first, I aim to highlight the links between macro-level social change and people's intimate, personal efforts to negotiate their identities as they grow older. My second, more abstract aim is to propose an alternative to the way that the life course is conceived of in the common imagination. The existing schema—which paints life as a temporal trip down a road or a lane—is perhaps most poetically conveyed in the opening lines of Dante's *Inferno*: "Midway along the journey of our life / I woke to find myself in some dark woods / for I had wandered off from the straight path." The notion that human life consists of a "straight path"—or any kind of path—from birth to death is a comforting one. It suggests that life's journey takes place on solid ground, and that we can find our way if we simply follow in the footsteps of those who came before us. But I will demonstrate here that retracing the steps of previous generations is not always possible, particularly for those who grow older amid historical ruptures. I suggest that a more apt metaphor for the aging process is a trip along a river: in the same way that one can't step into the same river twice, it is also impossible to travel down the same river twice. Each generation's journey is uniquely shaped by the sediments of history, by both natural and man-made changes in course, and by the mercurial ebbs and flows of policy.

The exact parameters of the *dama* persona may be subjective, but its origins can be traced to the concrete reality of demographic, economic, and social changes that rendered previous models of old age untenable or irrelevant. In other words, the middle-aged and older women who are identified as *dama* are not merely experimenting with hairstyles or hobbies like congregational dancing. Like many people around the globe who are aging in rapidly changing social landscapes, these women are trying to carve out new identities for themselves because they lack relatable or achievable ways of growing old. These attempts are not always well understood or met favorably by the Chinese public. Despite how much urban Chinese life has changed, gendered expectations that constrain women's abilities to live according to their own wishes have remained pervasive and, in some cases, have gained renewed traction in the post-reform era (Angeloff, Lieber, and Jayaram 2012; Liu 2011; Shea 2005). For older women, complicated gender politics are further compounded by shifting attitudes toward aging and the declining social status of elders in Chinese society (Yan 2003). Taken together, these conditions put women of this generational cohort—particularly those who deviate from socially sanctioned models of aging—at a distinct disadvantage.

In what follows, I examine how decades of dramatic social change have upended the aging process and produced new challenges and opportunities for people growing old in an unstable social landscape. I pay particular attention to how these changes have affected the behavior and attitudes of a generational cohort of urban Chinese women who received relatively few benefits from the country's rapid economic boom despite enduring the brunt of the accompanying social changes. I argue that aging has become a process that has become bound to—and complicated by—subjective personal choices as a result of recent economic reforms and subsequent changes in the social fabric.

Aging in the Midst of Social Change

Anthropologists have been concerned with variations in how societies treat different stages of the life course since the early days of the discipline. In her introduction to *Coming of Age in Samoa* ([1928] 1961), Margaret Mead tells us that the goal of her book is to answer a central question: "Are the disturbances which vex our adolescents due to the nature of adolescence itself or to the civilization? Under different conditions does adolescence present a different picture?" By "our adolescents," she meant Western ones in general and American ones in particular, whose tendencies toward psychological distress and rebellious behavior had already become taken for granted even though adolescence itself had only recently emerged as a distinct life stage in the late nineteenth century (Lesko 2012; Linders 2016). Among the contributions that *Coming of Age in Samoa* has made, one of its enduring legacies lies in the conceit that life stages are not necessarily tethered to biological age but are rather fluid categories subject to cultural influence. In other words, the aging process must be understood in the context of social processes.

While Mead challenges previously held assumptions about what occurs during adolescence, she does not question the existence of adolescence itself—or any other life stage—as stable objects of inquiry. This intervention came to the anthropology of the life course on the heels of the discipline's so-called reflexive turn (see Behar and Gordon 1995; Clifford and Marcus 1986; Ruby 1982), in works such as Lawrence Cohen's *No Aging in India* (1998) and Sarah Lamb's *White Saris and Sweet Mangos* (2000). Examining the emergence of new analytical categories of senility in postcolonial Indian society, Cohen contends that both Western biomedical paradigms and local cultural frameworks pathologized old age, ultimately arguing that both physical and mental processes of aging are "rooted in culture and political economy" (6). Similarly, Lamb articulates the ways in which cultural practices and changing notions of modernity figure into aging Bengali women's narratives of their own lives. Both books challenge the notion that old age is somehow insulated from or immune to broader social contexts. Lamb goes even further along this line of argumentation in a later work (2009) by asserting that older people cannot be assumed to embrace "traditional" ways of life universally or uncritically; people at all stages of the life course are capable of reflecting on and absorbing their present social environments, and therefore of becoming agents of social change. Like Lamb, I use "aging as a lens to explore how social worlds are constituted and taken apart" (Lamb 2000, 239). While there have been numerous studies detailing the practical implications of China's aging population, the scholarship on how demographic changes affect people's attitudes and outlooks on old age is still emerging.

Demographic Changes and the Transformation of Social Hierarchy

The first and most obvious way that old age has changed is increasing longevity. As was the case for much of human history, people in pre-industrial China were susceptible to childhood illness, maternal death, malnutrition, infectious disease, and other causes of early mortality. However, advancements in nutrition, medical care, and general standards of living have led to a dramatic increase in life expectancy: a person born in China in 1960, the first year that the World Bank began compiling data, could expect to live to age forty-four. A person born in 2016, in comparison, is expected to live to age seventy-six (World Bank 2018).

Nowadays, it is not unusual for Chinese urbanites to live into their eighties or nineties, and older people make up an increasingly large proportion of the overall population. To provide a concrete example, in the twenty-thousand-person urban community (*shequ*) where I conducted most of my fieldwork, there were approximately three thousand people over the age of sixty, one thousand people over the age of eighty, and six people over the age of one hundred in 2017 (interview with *shequ* officials June 8, 2017). This means that almost a quarter of the people living in the neighborhood were middle-aged or older. For another point of reference, all my dance group interlocutors—the majority of whom were in their sixties—had at least one parent or parent-in-law still living while I was in Chengdu conducting research.

These demographic shifts mean that people in their sixties, who may well have been considered elders a few generations ago, are now solidly middle-aged relative to the overall population. This would be significant in and of itself, but its effects have also been magnified by a seismic shift in China's age-based social hierarchy. Elder veneration is a mainstay of traditional Confucian ethics, and respecting elders remains a crucial element of the Chinese moral landscape. However, this moral foundation, which only a few generations ago had seemed so immutable, has shifted dramatically over the past century and continues to change.

To fully understand these changes, we need to take a step back to examine how social status—that is, the standards by which lives are appraised and measured—has shifted in recent years. The ethic of filial piety was set forth by Confucius and his disciple Zengzi in a work called the *Xiaojing* in the fourth century BC and has shaped social interactions throughout much of Chinese history (Baker 1979; Chin, Freedman, and Joint Committee 1970). This text, translated as *The Classic of Filial Piety*, outlines proper behavior between fathers and sons, husbands and wives, younger brothers and elder brothers, and rulers and subjects, arguing in each instance that the junior (or female) person in the relationship ought to defer to the senior one. In practical terms, this means that people venerated their ancestors and their elders, and that younger people deferred to the judgment of elders in all respects (Hsu 1967). However, filial piety was not just meant to be a guide for domestic relations. The hierarchical roles that are outlined in the *Xiaojing* are meant to serve as the foundation for an orderly, harmonious society.

Over the centuries and through numerous political movements that strengthened and codified the influence of Confucianism on Chinese society, filial piety played a major role in shaping ordinary people's attitudes about social hierarchy and what constitutes appropriate behavior. These attitudes ran so deeply that that when twentieth-century intellectuals—first during the New Culture Movement of 1911 and later during the Communist Revolution—set out to modernize Chinese culture, critiquing filial piety was among their first lines of attack. Leaders of both political movements believed that deference to elders hindered innovation and was the root cause of China's relative economic and technological stagnation. By the time Mao launched his Cultural Revolution in 1966, upending the age-based social hierarchy had become a cornerstone of his efforts to transform Chinese society: young people were encouraged to rebel against the old, and people who held positions of seniority were deposed in favor of younger (and more malleable) replacements.

Though these traumatic political campaigns undoubtedly set the stage for what was to come, perhaps nothing structurally dismantled the social status of elders more efficiently than the post-reform job market. Unlike the previous communist social contract under Mao in which urban residents were promised lifetime employment, reformer Deng Xiaoping's "socialism with Chinese characteristics" allowed for companies to compete for profit even if it meant letting go of less productive workers. No age discrimination law exists in the People's Republic, and the nature of the manufacturing jobs that were available during the earlier years of the economic boom meant that corporations desired young, able-bodied workers. Public-sector workers must also contend with compulsory retirement ages: sixty for men, and fifty-five and fifty for women in white- and blue-collar jobs, respectively. These policies created an environment where employers openly discriminate based on age. The overall effects of these reforms on the social landscape cannot be overstated: they transformed the social hierarchy such that those who managed to "get rich first" now occupied the top social strata rather than those with the most seniority in terms of age or rank. Though elder veneration is still a salient feature of contemporary Chinese cultural practices, the fact remains that elders have lost considerable social stature in recent decades.

These changes have been especially stark for women. Young women occupied the lowest stratum in the traditional Chinese social hierarchy, and a woman's life generally improved as she grew older. This remained the case until recent years. Though China's closed borders during the Mao era means that there is little ethnographic data to draw from during this period, we can look to studies from other sinophone contexts for insight. In her work in the Hong Kong New Territories in the 1970s, Rubie Watson (1986) asserts that a young girl's parents would have assumed that she would leave her birth family when she married, and thus may have withheld their resources accordingly. A bride would expect to live with her husband's family, where she would perform the lion's share of domestic tasks and where mistreatment from her mother-in-law was a distinct possibility. Her situation would improve only when she gave birth to children of her own and rose through the ranks of the household hierarchy (Parish and Whyte 1978). By mid-age, she may have finally earned the respect of her in-laws and carved out a life of her own, possibly even with her own daughters-in-law to bully. Margery Wolf (1972) famously noted the stark difference between the "terrified young bride" and the "confident, often lewd old woman who has outlived her mother-in-law and her husband," and argued that the happiest, most secure years of a woman's life were those at the end of her life course. When one compares this expected life trajectory to that of Qingyi's, whose life history is outlined in the previous chapter and who contended with destabilizing political campaigns in her youth, lost her job and sense of personal identity in mid-age, and who is growing old in an uncertain social landscape, one can easily see how much has changed.

As remarkable as these transformations have been, their impacts are further exacerbated by concurrent shifts in how personal identity is construed in post-reform China. In the agrarian villages in which most Chinese people lived before the previous century, personhood was not something endowed at birth but rather something that a person earns by accomplishing a series of appropriate tasks at the proper time. It is through this process of *zuoren,* or what Yunxiang Yan (2017) has translated to "doing personhood," that an individual becomes him or herself. Marriage, children, and establishing a home were prerequisites to being considered a full person. In such a social context, elders were addressed by kinship terms like *daye* (grandfather or elder uncle) or *daniang* (elder aunt), and addressing someone by these terms was a signifier of respect. In other words, the traditional Chinese model of personhood differs significantly from the "ageless self" that Sharon Kaufman (1986) analyzes in her book of the same title. Whereas the American elders in Kaufman's study coped with the changes associated with aging by maintaining continuous—and ageless—senses of individual identity, personhood in the traditional Chinese context was age-graded by definition and by practice.

Seen in this light, the Confucian ethic of filial piety and the obligation to respect elders take on an additional layer of meaning: elders were not simply revered for the sake of custom, but rather because they were morally superior since they had accomplished more of life's tasks. They were more deserving of respect than those who were still in the process of becoming full persons. In post-reform society, however, people no longer have a sense of shared social identity or agreed-upon models of personhood. Xin Liu (2002) argues that people now live out their lives as "characters," like "boss" or "young miss." In the absence of a unifying point on the moral horizon toward which people can aim, Liu conceives of contemporary Chinese society as a performance in which each individual actor struggles to tell her own story without a clear script. Erving Goffman (1959) would argue that these social performances comprise the basis of all social interactions, but their efficacy in traditional settings would have been constrained by the rigid social hierarchy that limited the extent to which people could assert their identities as individuals.

I do not wish to go so far as to suggest that people did not participate in social performances aimed at guiding others' impressions of them prior to the social changes I outlined in the previous pages. It is also true that many aspects of traditional customs remain in place. I will never forget one of my mother's local friends—upon hearing that I intended to do research on retirement and aging—admonishing me, "Never call anyone *daye* [grandfather]! If you want to talk to an old guy, call him *dage* [older brother] instead." Her meaning was plain: older men do not want to be seen as grandfathers by young women, and flattering them by addressing them as "older brother" will make them more likely to answer questions. After all, terms of address are laden with social significance in China, and calling someone the wrong thing can lead to misunderstanding or awkwardness. To put this another way, identity—and age-graded identity in particular—is still determined at least in part by external recognition. My own realization that I was crossing the boundary into adulthood came when, at the age of seventeen, I was introduced to a family friend's toddler as *ayi* ("auntie") rather than *jiejie* ("older sister"). A few years later, people in their sixties or seventies became "aunties" and "uncles," rather than "grandmother" and "grandfather," and my adult status became increasingly cemented in the process.

But continuity and change are not mutually exclusive. Numerous scholars of China have noted (see Lei 2003) that the social changes of the past half-century have made it more possible for people to manage their outward presentations according to their own feelings or circumstances rather than according to social custom. For people in late middle age, this means having to figure out aspects of the aging process for themselves.

Old age is not the only axis of identity undergoing a process of reinterpretation, but these broader changes in the organizing mechanisms of Chinese society have given people increased freedom to assert their personal wishes about how to be old, as well as increased confusion about what being old now means. When analyzed through this context, it becomes clear that the *dama* persona can be understood as a manifestation of Chinese women's efforts to seek out new or alternative ways of being older. Seen in this light, the *dama* persona is one of Xin Liu's "characters"—a response to the receding relevance of previous models of aging that do not fit any recognizable models of old age precisely because the guideposts for what a life trajectory ought to look like have changed so much.

When afforded the leeway to reimagine old age, what sorts of aesthetics, attitudes, and activities do urban Chinese women embrace? Growing older is a profoundly confusing enterprise for many women in urban China due to a lack of clear expectations about how the process should unfold, but with this confusion also comes an opportunity to incorporate vivid colors, outspoken personal expression, and uninhibited camaraderie with other women in their age cohort into their lives.

"I Don't Know What I Am"

When I was a child growing up in Chengdu in the 1980s and 1990s, there was very little variation in how a woman over age sixty looked. She invariably wore dark-colored clothing in the "Mao Suit" style, consisting of cotton or woolen trousers and a jacket cut generously so as to hang loosely from the body. Her shoes were black canvas with white rubber soles. Her hair—never dyed and in various shades of gray—was either chin-length and swept out of her face with bobby pins or pulled back into a tight coif at the base of her neck. If she wore any jewelry, it would be simple and sentimental adornments like enamel pins or a ring. She wore no makeup. High heels were out of the question.

I remember all of the older women I knew, including both of my own grandmothers, looking like this throughout my childhood. When I was deeply concerned with my own apparel during my teenage years, I once asked my maternal grandmother why she still wore the same clothes as she did in the "old times" despite the fact that there were so many more options. She replied that it was a matter of habit: women her age, she explained, spent their younger days laboring at work and at home. It was also a time during which focusing on appearances was associated with bourgeois or counterrevolutionary attitudes; wearing something eye-catching was a sure way to earn a bad reputation. And when fashions began to change at the onset of economic reforms—well, by then they were no longer interested in trying to keep up. Now in her nineties and with her perennial woolen trousers and short hair, my maternal grandmother looks very much the part of the typical "old woman" that exists in my and other Chinese people's imaginations.

So when I met the exuberant Ms. Liu at a dance group social gathering and she told me that she did not think of herself as an "old person," I knew exactly what she meant. "I just don't feel old," she said, "and I don't think I look old either." Ms. Liu is a high school classmate of Rui, one of my key interlocutors. Ms. Liu belongs to a dance group herself, and like most women who

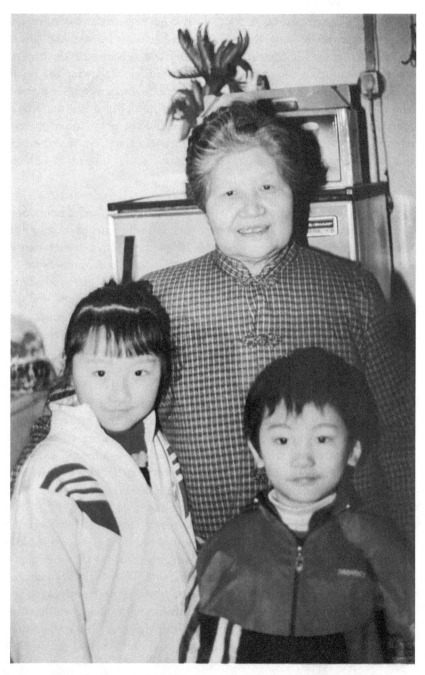

FIGURE 4 The author's maternal grandmother, ca. age sixty-five, with the author and the author's cousin in the mid-1990s. (Photo courtesy of author's mother)

participate in congregational dancing, she is in her early sixties. Ms. Liu was a young woman when Deng Xiaoping initiated reforms in 1978 and subsequently lost her job when her state-owned employer privatized at the turn of the millennium. She also spent the years immediately following the layoff feeling listless before eventually finding camaraderie among a group of women who had many of the same experiences. They danced, dined, and socialized together. Over time, Ms. Liu and her friends (whom she affectionately referred to as her "sisters") formed a tight-knit social group that shared everything from commiseration about conflicts with adult children to fashion advice.

At the dinner party where we met, Ms. Liu was elegantly dressed in a flowing magenta calf-length dress layered over leggings and low-heeled boots. She had soft bangs that just brushed the top of her carefully penciled brows while the rest of her sleek dyed-auburn hair was pulled into a ponytail and fastened with an ornate hair clip. Though she was somewhat taller than the other women at the dinner and multiple people complimented her on her figure, Ms. Liu's fashion sense was far from unusual among dance group participants, and she fit right in with the women from the dance group. Despite her statement about not feeling old, Ms. Liu shared numerous thoughts and fears about the aging process with me when she learned about my research: the horror of seeing your face change before your eyes, the anxiety of hearing about once-vibrant friends becoming ill, the panic that can set in when you feel your body slowing down. "Even a small cut heals so slowly now," she complained. The inherent contradiction in her attitudes on old age was not lost on her: she did not feel old, and yet she experienced and contended with the symptoms of aging in her everyday life. "Getting old," she remarked about her own confusion, "is not so simple." I told her about what my grandmother had shared with me when I was a teen. Maybe, I ventured, she did not feel old because she did not resemble what she thought old women were supposed to look like.

At this, Ms. Liu emitted a literal squeal of recognition. "YES! That is exactly right! People my age looked so old when I was young. They also acted so old." She went on to paint a mental picture of old age even more vivid and certainly more geriatric than my own: a wizened crone with yellowing teeth that prevented her from chewing, a humped back that prevented her from looking up, an unsteady gait that prevented her from venturing out from her familiar surroundings, and, most of all, an imperious, self-righteous air. This unflattering portrait did not resemble Ms. Liu in any way. "Now that I am that age myself," she concluded, "I don't know what I am."

Ms. Liu's confession may strike the average Chinese person as strange. For most ordinary observers, there is no question about what Ms. Liu is—she is a *dama*. Everything about her outward presentation, from her clothes to her comportment to her choice of friends and social activities, marks her as such. In

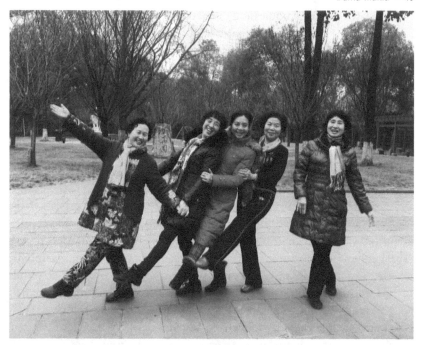

FIGURE 5 A group of women in their early sixties, including the author's aunt (center), posing together in a Chengdu park in 2017. The women are members of a dance group and self-identify as *dama*. They are donning typical *dama* permed, dyed hair as well as brightly colored clothing and scarves. (Photo by Claudia Huang)

later conversations, Ms. Liu even told me that she does not mind the label and occasionally refers to herself and her friends as *dama* in social media posts. But the fact remains that Ms. Liu harbors doubt and uncertainty about who she is becoming as she grows older, and my research indicates that she is in good company. My interlocutors frequently expressed similar ambivalence and even defiance about their age-graded and gendered identities. "I'm old now, yes," another interlocutor named Yun once remarked while we were discussing her decision to take a series of glamour shots at a local photography studio, "but why should I limit myself to doing 'old lady things' [*laoniang dongxi*]?"

The fact that aging women in contemporary China are rejecting the bland woolen trousers of their mothers' generation in favor of brighter colors and greater attention to personal appearance is not, in itself, remarkable. Scholars of China have long observed that the post-reform "consumer revolution" (Davis 2000) produced new consumer desires, which in turn created novel forms of gendered subjectivity and self-cultivation (Rofel 2007). Writing on the rise of grooming and beautification industries, Claudia Liebelt (2016) argues that the conditions of late capitalism in Chinese society give women little choice but to make new "gendered bodies and moral selves" (9). Jie Yang (2011) stakes out a similar claim when she notes that the post-reform market economy capitalizes on women for their labor as well as their consumption; women are pressured into seeking aesthetic remedies from the emerging beauty industry, which is in turn staffed by low-paid women workers. There is no doubt that Ms. Liu, Yun, or any other colorfully attired older woman in urban China has been influenced by these developments. However, the point I wish to make is not the mere fact that women identified as *dama* are refashioning themselves in a new mold, but rather how their chosen mold can complicate the preexisting frameworks that are commonly used to think about aging, gender, and personhood in post-reform China.

It would be difficult to make sense of the *dama* aesthetic and persona if one were to rely on the analytical categories that scholars have devised to investigate the status of women in post-reform society. For example, Sally McWilliams (2012) argues that a "dyad of femininities" emerged out of China's economic transformation: the first is a bride in a Western wedding gown, which stands in for a worldly, romantic feminine ideal, and the second is a young woman in a Chinese *qipao*, which represents a sexualized version of the traditional cultured lady. While these two idealized womanhoods are distinct from one another, they both emphasize youth and sexual attractiveness. Jie Yang (2011) addresses the aging process in her discussion of the resurgence of sexual difference and hierarchy in Chinese society, but she focuses her analysis on the growing bifurcation between the young and the old. In the opening paragraphs of her article, Yang introduces the story of a woman in her fifties who seeks out cosmetic surgery to re-entice (and seek revenge against) her unfaithful husband. This woman, Yang argues, is trapped in a gendered discourse that divides women into "tender women [*nennü*]" and "ripe women [*shunü*]"—a dichotomy that is promoted by market forces and the Chinese state in order to highlight sexual differences and encourage consumer spending.

Women who identify as *dama* are certainly not immune to these discourses, and there is evidence that the desire to appear youthful informs some of their aesthetic choices. I once stepped into an elevator with a half-dozen women from a dance group and was struck by the fact that every single person was dressed in pink or fuchsia. In response to my observation, someone explained that colorful clothing compensated for the loss of bloom in their complexions. And yet, it would be wrong to conclude that women who identify as *dama* are modeling themselves after either of the femininities presented in McWilliams's analytical dyad. The typical *dama* look is resolutely feminine without pretention or reference to romance and sexuality. There are, of course, variations between individuals, but something like a codified *dama* style has nonetheless emerged. According to one popular Chinese website, it consists of "batwing tops, flared pants, sunglasses, straw hats, and silk scarves" ("中国大码" 2020).

In my own observations, women in this demographic also tend to prefer permed and dyed hair (usually in shades of auburn) and penciled-in eyebrows paired with an otherwise bare face. It is a look that is full of contradictions: it is neither youthful nor geriatric (according to customary cultural norms), carefully considered but not exactly fashionable, immediately recognizable yet difficult to pin down. I also found little evidence to support the notion that women who identify as *dama* manage their appearances or behaviors to appeal to their husbands (or any other men, for that matter.) When I playfully asked Yun what her husband thought of her glamour shots, for example, she scoffed and replied that she had not bothered to show them to him. They were, however, shared widely among her friends. And while posing for photos is an important pastime for women in this demographic (a selfie stick is another indispensable accessory in the *dama* uniform), the resulting photographs serve as tokens of friendship rather than displays of vanity. When I sent photos from a dance group performance to an interlocutor, she excitedly posted them to the group WeChat, writing, "Sisters, I hope that we may look back on these photos as we grow old as a reminder of the exciting days we shared together."

In this chapter, I have examined the emergence of a new category of aged person known as *dama* and argued that its existence complicates both traditional and market-driven frameworks of identity in the People's Republic of China. The *dama* persona reflects a complex embodiment of both femininity and old age—born out of the shared experiences of a particular generation—that defies existing analytical categories. The concrete realities of a longer lifespan and a transformed social order have unsettled the ways in which people perceive and experience the aging process; as people grow older in a changing society, old age itself becomes a moving target. It is no wonder, then, that my friend Xia can confidently declare that you "know [a *dama*] when you see one," but a woman who is so clearly a *dama* such as Ms. Liu can express confusion about who and what she is. It may be many years before the *dama* persona finds a secure place in the cultural lexicon, and it is possible that some new stereotype or persona will arise in the interim to supplant the *dama* in the popular imagination. In the meantime, retired Chinese women are demonstrating that what they choose to wear, do, and spend time with has broad implications for how old age is perceived and experienced in Chinese society.

The New Old Age

When I was doing preliminary fieldwork in the summers of 2014 and 2015, I approached as many dance groups as possible on the streets of Chengdu to speak to participants about their experiences. Many of them also had questions for me, the most common of which was, "How old do you think I am?"

It would be posed less as a sincere question and more as a challenge. I sensed from the start that the point of this exchange was for them to correct my guess, and I mastered the game before long: no matter how old I thought the asker was, I would reply "fifty-eight," because most dancers were older than that. Almost invariably, I would be corrected with a tone of triumph—"I'm actually sixty-five!" "You're wrong! I'm sixty-two!"—at which point I would express surprise and congratulate her on her youthful appearance. I must have played this game dozens, if not hundreds, of times. Though I knew its rules, I struggled to understand the rationale behind the game: why bother making yourself look younger if you are going to reveal your true age anyway? The game finally began to make more sense when I thought about it in the social context in which these women were growing older. There are certainly still limits to an individual's control over how she will be perceived, as the episode with the woman on the bus at the beginning of this chapter reveals, but there is also more space for personal exploration. By setting up a playful exchange in which their "real" ages are the punchline, these women are striking a delicate balance between managing their personal appearance to suit their own preferences, on the one hand, and acknowledging the continuing importance of external validation, on the other. In this sense, they have also mastered the game.

Old age is undergoing a period of profound transformation in the People's Republic of China. This transformation is also part of a much larger global phenomenon. Many societies are rapidly aging, and neoliberal policies that emphasize personal responsibility in the aging process have also produced commensurate desires to grow old on one's own terms. For example, in a story that received international media attention in 2018, a man named Emile Ratelband from the Netherlands petitioned his government to officially change his age from sixty-nine to forty-nine. His reasons for wanting this change were rooted in practical desires: he told reporters that if he were forty-nine, he could attract more employers and receive more attention from younger women on online dating apps. Besides, he said, his doctor told him that he was as healthy as a man in his forties. The justification he presented to the courts, however, was more philosophical in nature. "[Americans and Europeans] are free people," he explained to a reporter from the *Washington Post*. "We can make our own decisions if we want to change our name, or if we want to change our gender. So I want to change my age. My feeling about my body and about my mind is that I'm about 40 or 45" (Stanley-Becker 2018). Unfortunately for Mr. Ratelband, the Dutch courts disagreed: they ruled that while Mr. Ratelband was "at liberty to feel 20 years younger than his real age and act accordingly," a person's age actually has a number of legal and social implications and therefore cannot be amended based on personal whim (Domonoske 2018).

Few people living in China have the liberty to share Mr. Ratelband's sanguine attitudes about the superior power of personal choice over state authority (a fact that Ratelband himself acknowledges by specifically naming the United States and Europe in his statement to reporters). However, the Dutch man's efforts to change his age and his government's denial of these efforts nonetheless mirrors the renegotiation of the aging process taking place in China today. Women who identify as *dama* are not formally petitioning to change their ages, but their very existence serves as a reminder that it is possible for the aging process to take unexpected turns. In rapidly changing societies, the material conditions that make certain ideals of old age possible may vanish on the horizon, leaving people no choice but to reimagine what it means to be old and adapt their ideals accordingly. For many urban Chinese women, customary models of becoming a revered matriarch in old age have been made nearly impossible to achieve due to economic reforms, the one-child policy, and the rise of an increasingly youth-centric consumer culture. However, these same changes have also offered them the chance to dance for leisure, to wear colorful clothing, and to spend time with their friends.

Unlike Mr. Ratelband, the women in the Dancing Beauties and the Sunset Dance Group have no delusions of grandeur with respect to the limits of self-determination. Though they do not emulate the traditional trappings of old age modeled by earlier generations and largely do not participate in the youth-focused beauty industry, most are nevertheless aware that their efforts to create a new kind of old age strike some others as ridiculous. For now, they seem unbothered, choosing to focus instead on their own relationships and experiences.

This does not mean, however, that the *dama* persona is superficial or that its sphere of influence is limited to those who directly participate. To the contrary: the efforts of women who identify as *dama* to grow older on their own terms and in a manner that is consistent with their present social contexts has significant ramifications for Chinese society. By creating a gendered aesthetic of aging that reflects and responds to their generational experiences, these women are challenging others to reimagine what old age can look like and feel like. It is true that their way of growing older may not continue to resonate over time—I would be surprised if middle-aged and older women still dyed their hair auburn or danced together in groups in another thirty or fifty years—but the *dama* have demonstrated that it is possible to chart a new course on life's journey. When younger people imagine their older selves, there is now a greater range of possibility in their minds' eye.

As China's population continues to grow older and as the country continues to gain economic and political strength, further changes to the aging process seem all but certain—but remain to be seen. What is beyond question, however, is that women who are identified as *dama* have opened a conversation about the gendered aesthetics of old age that will undoubtedly continue for some time.

3
Families under (Peer) Pressure

Retired women living in urban China must contend with a fundamental tension in their lives: on the one hand, they are freer than ever before to live their lives on their own terms; on the other hand, expectations that older women devote themselves to their families remain salient in Chinese society and can become especially intense as these women become grandmothers. For women who participate in common-interest social groups like congregational dance groups, an additional layer of complications may arise as they struggle to balance these two diametrically opposed forces. Dance groups are almost entirely made up of people who come together of their own volition to pursue their personal interests. With the small exception of some groups that are formed by community officials, urban dance groups are almost entirely self-organized. These groups are, in essence, held together by the participants' desires to engage in self-cultivation and to spend time on relationships and hobbies of their own choosing. This means that when any one person chooses to honor her family obligations over her own interests, including dancing, others in the dance group are also affected.

This chapter examines the uneasy balance that retired women try to strike when confronted with the tensions between self-interest and morally laden family obligations in post-reform urban China as well as how friendships figure into this fraught calculus. Most of urban China's *dama* belong to the so-called sandwich generation (see Zhang and Goza 2006; Tu 2016) and perform the lion's share of caregiving duties in their families. In addition to often being expected to care for their grandchildren, many also have elderly parents and parents-in-law who require attention and resources. The result, as scholars have noted, is widespread exhaustion and stress associated with caregiving among women in this age cohort (Chen, Liu, and Mair 2011; Goh 2011). Further complicating matters is the fact that the relative social status of middle-aged and elderly women has declined in recent years. While elders—and grandmothers would have certainly been counted as elders—commanded a great deal of respect in traditional Chinese kinship hierarchies, the gravitational center of Chinese families has recently begun to shift away from elders and toward young children (Fong 2002; Kipnis 2009; Yan 2016).

All this is to say that the tide has shifted against Chinese elders, and people in the sandwich generation have plenty to complain about. Their current predicament can be traced to the numerous changes in the traditional family structure that have occurred since the middle of the past century, including Chinese Communist Party policies that destabilized patriarchal authority as well as pressures from the market economy that rendered traditional family structures untenable (Davis and Harrell 1993; Yan 2003; Santos and Harrell 2016). None of these changes have made the bonds of kinship insignificant. They have, however, introduced new challenges to family cohesion as well as emerging opportunities for individual family members to negotiate their relationships with one another.

The nature, content, and stakes of these negotiations are the focus of this chapter. Erin Thomason (2021) has argued that long-suffering grandparents in rural areas invoke their misery as their contribution to their families; without the ability to offer their children financial support and without the means to support themselves in later life if they do not receive care from these same children, they have no choice but to frame the indignity of their present situations as necessary sacrifices made on the altar of family solidarity. The situation is markedly different in urban areas. Though retired urban women echo many of the same complaints about inverted family dynamics, their relative financial independence from their children (due to high rates of home ownership and monthly pension payments from their former public-sector employers) allow them more options to navigate the trend of descending familism that is experienced by all Chinese elders.

Given their relatively privileged circumstances, many urban retirees have the option to prioritize personal interests over family obligations, particularly if they believe their family dynamics are too heavily skewed to their disadvantage. I have argued elsewhere (Huang 2016) that women who participate in congregational dance groups use these groups as vehicles for self-expression and as places where they can carve out meaningful lives on their own terms. But because this self-cultivation takes place within a collective enterprise, the demands of personal interest and friendship are closely interlinked.

In a society where putting one's family before one's own personal interests is still widely considered the morally righteous course of action, choosing to honor one's own concerns over those of one's family requires the support, validation, and in some cases forceful persuasion from one's friends. In other words, in order for these women to live lives of their own, they must stick together.

While the study of kinship has a long tradition in anthropology, the literature on friendship is considerably thinner. According to scholars such as Pitt-Rivers (1973) and Carrier (1999), this relative oversight can be attributed to an often-held assumption that kinship ties are permanent, universal, and compulsory, whereas friendships are ephemeral, idiosyncratic, and voluntary. There have been a few notable studies that challenge these assumptions by highlighting the ways in which solidarity among friends not only can be important for mitigating risks and creating social cohesion, but in some cases are even crucial for survival (see Abrahams 1999; Gratz 2004; Santos-Granero 2007). The retired women who participate in congregational dance groups are not grappling for survival. They are, however, engaged in a struggle to maintain their senses of self while inhabiting the bottom tier of the family hierarchy. Even though the friendships I examine in this chapter vary in terms of closeness and intensity, they are all, as Jane Dyson (2010) would say, settings for social production because, for those people who participate in them, they function as avenues for self-preservation or self-improvement.

This chapter looks at four cases that showcase just how tensions between family duties and individual interests can collide for retired urban women who are grandmothers, focusing on how their friendships are interwoven into these already complex situations. The first case demonstrates the ways in which congregational dancers use social pressure to bully a group member who, according to the group's estimation, spends too much time and energy tending to her family duties. The second case further illuminates how much dance groups rely on the participants' continued commitment to the group and how the group dynamics may be threatened when participants have other priorities. In the third case, I zero in on two friends whose very different styles of managing the aforementioned tensions between self-interest and family duty threaten to come between them. Finally, the fourth case focuses on how grandmothers' willingness (or lack thereof) to provide childcare can figure into young couples' plans to expand their families. I conclude with some conjectures about where these rumblings of discontent might lead and the implications of the greater emphasis on personal happiness in the family lives of Chinese urban retirees.

Bullying Qiu

The Dancing Beauties held its annual end-of-year party at an upscale karaoke bar in one of Chengdu's ritziest neighborhoods. Karaoke in China is perhaps best known as an evening activity for groups of young professionals and businessmen; deals are negotiated between rounds of singing, and young female hostesses lubricate the conversation with ample amounts of liquor. But at two o'clock in the afternoon, when private rooms are available at an early-bird discount, karaoke bars are havens for retirees who wish to belt out songs from revolutionary-era films and pop singles from the 1980s and 1990s. Afternoon karaoke was a favorite pastime of the Dancing Beauties, and on this occasion, the group's de-facto leader, Teacher Yuan, booked a private room with money left over from the group's membership dues. On the appointed day and time, the group met in the lobby and made its way to the second floor, where private rooms lined both sides of a long, brightly lit corridor.

Everyone was settling in with the usual greetings, snacks, and song selections when a woman whom I had never seen before walked into the room. She was short-statured, with auburn hair, and looked to be in her late fifties. She glanced around a little nervously before someone spotted her and ran toward the door where she stood, shouting greetings along the way. She was soon mobbed by nearly everyone in the room. Someone asked her if she had lost weight. Someone else complimented her on her purple sweater. Everyone wanted to know how the baby was. I was left sitting alone in the far corner, utterly confused by the fact that this seeming stranger was being treated like an old friend. By that time, I had already been a member of the Dancing Beauties for four months. Though some people attended the dance practices only sporadically, it did not seem possible that I could have completely overlooked someone. The mystery was short-lived. I soon learned that the newcomer was actually a four-year veteran of the group named Qiu. Her son and daughter-in-law had welcomed their first child less than two weeks prior to my arrival in Chengdu, and Qiu had been away because she had taken on full-time caregiving duties for her infant grandchild.

I was not the only one who found Qiu's seemingly abrupt reappearance to the dance group's social scene noteworthy. As the afternoon wore on and people took turns singing their karaoke selections, Qiu fielded a number of questions—some of them quite pointed—about why she had failed to keep in touch during her absence and why she had been away for so long. She demurred on most of the questions, claiming that she was simply too busy to keep up with the online group chats and was too tired to come to the dance classes. Her friends did not let her off the hook so easily. As the karaoke session concluded and the group made its way to a nearby restaurant for dinner, group members continued to harangue her about how she was handling her transition into grandmotherhood.

It was apparent from the start that Qiu prioritized maintaining good relations with her son and daughter-in-law. It became clear that most of the other women interpreted Qiu's devotion to her son's new nuclear family as a weakness or even a sense of capitulation. "When is your daughter-in-law going to let you have your next night off?" a group member named Jiaming asked as we sat down to eat. Her thinly veiled suggestion that Qiu was at the mercy of her daughter-in-law—a direct reversal of the customary hierarchy in traditional Chinese families—caused quite a stir around the table. Several of the women chuckled and even clapped, and everyone directed glances at Qiu to see how she would respond. Qiu laughed along but did not answer. The teasing reached a peak when, at the end of the meal, Qiu ordered extra portions of food to bring home for the young couple. "Oh, you are such an obedient mother-in-law!" exclaimed a normally soft-spoken group member named Yun. Again, everyone at the table burst into laughter. Perhaps because it had come from the gentle-tempered Yun, or perhaps because the comment was particularly barbed, Qiu's shoulders dropped and her cheeks became engulfed in a deep blush. The term Yun had used for "obedient" was *ting hua*, literally translated as "listen to words" [of authority]. It is a term that is often used when praising young children for good behavior (see Xu 2017), but it is never used to refer to an adult without some sense of irony or deprecation as the subtext.

For the first time that day, Qiu attempted to defend herself: she explained that her son and daughter-in-law loved the type of food served at the restaurant but had not had a chance to enjoy it since the baby's arrival. Unfortunately, this explanation only added fuel to the fire. Several people laughed, and someone pointedly jeered, "look at you being so filial!" Again, by "praising" Qiu in a manner usually reserved for children (after all, filial piety is defined as respect for one's elders), the women in the group aimed to draw attention to Qiu's (from their perspective) transgressive behavior and to shame her for it.

It is crucial to note that although the women in the Dancing Beauties invoked the language and norms of the traditional family hierarchy and used them as rhetorical weapons, they were not trying to enforce these norms. On the contrary, by taunting and insulting Qiu for her devotion to her family, they were building solidarity in an effort to establish new norms—norms that do not take a grandmother's financial and emotional resources for granted. This was a feat that they could not accomplish as individuals. The group's overt cruelty toward Qiu can be explained by the fact that Qiu was crossing the picket line, so to speak, by continuing to make sacrifices on behalf of her adult children. As the women's reactions to Qiu's relatively compliant disposition toward her son and daughter-in-law demonstrate, there was significant social pressure to show one's willingness to "fight back" against the inverted family dynamics.

But it turned out that Qiu had given more thought to the inherent tensions in her situation than her friends had given her credit for. At the end of the evening, Teacher Yuan suggested that Qiu and I catch the bus together since we happened to live in the same part of town. Under the increased scrutiny of her friends and group-mates, Qiu had been good-natured but cagey, rarely adding more than a few words to any exchange for fear that the conversation might turn on her. It was only after we sat down on the bus that Qiu started speaking with me candidly. At my gentle urging, she revealed that she longed to return to the group and that although she adored her grandson, she resented that he kept her from participating in her own social life. She even admitted that she was glad that the end was in sight: her daughter-in-law's six months of maternity leave would soon be over, after which the baby would be sent to live with the daughter-in-law's parents in another city, thus releasing Qiu from her caregiving duties.

Qiu is hardly alone in her ambivalence: confusion and doubt seem to be the primary emotions among many women with whom I spoke about the choice between taking care of their grandchildren and enjoying their retirement on their own terms. They are all too aware of the inverted power dynamics in the family, and they must weigh their own wishes against the risks of displeasing their adult children. Whereas Qiu made major social sacrifices to take care of her grandson, in her mind there would have been even greater repercussions had she refused: her daughter-in-law would have had to stay with her own parents for the duration of her maternity leave unless Qiu had agreed to care for the infant in Chengdu. By all accounts, Qiu got along quite well with her son and daughter-in-law, and it is unlikely that they were intentionally taking advantage of her. Nevertheless, they put her in the situation of having to choose between giving up her social life for six months or giving up the chance to bond with her infant grandson. Throughout our thirty-minute conversation, Qiu alternated between saying that she was looking forward to resuming her regular activities and that she was dreading the day when she would be separated from her grandchild.

Despite the relentless onslaught of not entirely good-humored taunting, the women in the Dancing Beauties stopped short of asking Qiu to abdicate her grandmotherly responsibilities in favor of spending more time with the group. Though at some point every woman asked her when she would be able to come dance again, no one pressed her to take time off from her childcare duties or offered her any practical suggestions on how she could get away from the family. Nevertheless, the group's prodding was clearly meant to send the message that Qiu's behavior was unacceptable. Moreover, by casting Qiu in a childlike position in their pointed jokes about filial piety and obedience, the group members were also seeking to undermine Qiu's sense of personal autonomy and to impress upon her that she would not receive the group's support until she demonstrated that she could assert her independence from her son, his wife, and her grandchild. The result was that at the end of the evening, Qiu was more conflicted than ever about how to balance her duties to her family, to her dance group, and to herself.

Committing to Teacher Yuan

A few weeks after the end-of-year karaoke party, Teacher Yuan told the Dancing Beauties that her son was expecting a child with his fiancée, due in late spring. The announcement immediately threw everyone into a panic. People assumed that Teacher Yuan would cancel dance classes for an indefinite amount of time after the baby's arrival. Teacher Yuan took great joy in correcting this assumption. "Not only will I keep teaching classes," she proclaimed, "I have also signed up for both the singing class and the African drum class at Old Age University during the summer term!" When incredulous group members asked how she planned to balance these activities with her caregiving duties, Teacher Yuan replied that the two sets of grandparents (meaning herself and her future daughter-in-law's parents) would take turns caring for the baby. "It's unreasonable to expect me to drop everything," she explained. "I have my own life to live, you know!" At this, the group enthusiastically praised Teacher Yuan for her independent attitude, and a few women who did not yet have a grandchild vowed to emulate her when their time came.

Teacher Yuan is intensely dedicated to the Dancing Beauties and leads it with the precision and iron will of a military commander. Not only does she teach the group's weekly dance classes, but she also single-handedly manages the group's finances, sets its agendas, and makes announcements via WeChat. I admit I was skeptical that Teacher Yuan would be able to follow through on her intentions after the baby arrived, but she proved me wrong. Her granddaughter was born in early May, and the dance classes resumed after a brief two-week hiatus. Teacher Yuan attended the courses at the old age university as planned, and in early July she even organized a group day trip to the countryside to pick peaches.

As it turned out, the group was threatened not by Teacher Yuan's family commitments but rather by her disappointment in the other members' inability to match her dedication to the group. In late September, a few hours before the afternoon dance class was scheduled to begin, the Dancing Beauties' WeChat group was flooded with messages from people excusing themselves from attendance due to various scheduling conflicts and illnesses. A few people usually excuse themselves each week, but this week had an unusual number of absences. It soon became clear that most of the class would not be in attendance. Teacher Yuan remained silent while people were sending their regrets and excuses, but just a few minutes prior to the start of the class she finally replied: "It looks like everyone is quite busy. After this semester is over, we will no longer hold this dance class."

When I arrived a few minutes late to the dance studio where the classes were held, I saw that there were only five people present—a very low turnout. Teacher Yuan made no mention of the absences and carried on as usual. No one spoke of the ominous WeChat announcement until the class had ended. As we filed out of the studio building and into the parking lot, Jiaming gently approached Teacher Yuan, who had headed straight for her electric scooter and was busy stuffing her belongings into the front basket. "Please give us another chance," Jiaming began. "I'll go home and tell the others that they have to stop taking breaks for no good reason." The rest of us gathered around. "I'll tell them to respect your time more," Jiaming continued as Teacher Yuan fussed with her scooter, pretending not to hear. "You take such pains with us! It's not right that they don't come." At this, Teacher Yuan finally looked up and began airing some of her long-held grievances. "It's not that I don't want to teach the class anymore," she complained. "It's that people really don't seem to have the time. I don't know why they don't have the time! I had to bathe my granddaughter before I came! And I still made it here on time!"

All of us gathered around her scooter agreed that it should not be so difficult to make a commitment for just a few hours per week, but Teacher Yuan was not satisfied. "I have never taken a break, you know! I have never a missed class, never! In all these years!" Jiaming agreed: "Yes, Sister Yuan," she said, switching to an affectionate term of address. "*Ni zhen xinku le*" [You really have worked so hard/suffered so much]. And in the future if you need to take a break, just let us know!" Teacher Yuan, however, was entirely immune to their entreaties. She declared that we could all still be friends, and that she would organize get-togethers occasionally so that everyone could stay in touch.

Later in the evening, Jiaming wrote a long message to the WeChat group thanking Teacher Yuan for her generous guidance, pledging that everyone will work harder in the future and begging Teacher Yuan to continue leading the classes. Others, including those who had been absent, soon chimed in. Most people offered similar assurances that things would be different going forward, but a few went even further. Someone posted an appointment confirmation for an optometry visit. Someone else posted a photo of a thermometer showing a feverish temperature. Yun wrote a lengthy explanation that she had been recruited for a *qipao* (a type of traditional Chinese dress) modeling competition and that against her wishes the organizers had scheduled rehearsals that day. She shared the rehearsal schedule, emphatically adding that she hated missing class. It was only when Ying, one of the group's most dedicated participants, wrote to say that her husband was in the hospital with appendicitis and expressed her regrets for her absence that Teacher Yuan finally broke her silence: "I know about your husband, Ying! You should take care of yourself too!"

After several more days of intermittent pleading, Teacher Yuan finally relented. The Dancing Beauties continued to hold weekly classes at the dance studio. However, the short-lived episode not only provided further proof that dance groups demand loyalty and commitment from their members, but also revealed the internal logic of how the members' loyalties are assessed and enforced. It is noteworthy that Teacher Yuan made a big deal about not allowing her new granddaughter to take precedence over the dance group, and she broke her silence only upon hearing of Ying's husband's illness. Over the course of the year that I spent with them, I slowly learned that there was a hierarchy of excuses for missing class among the women: taking care of grandchildren was seen as the least legitimate reason, choosing to honor another personal commitment (such as Yun's *qipao* competition) was somewhere in the middle, and skipping class for a spouse or parent's illness was universally accepted and supported. For example, though the group chastised Qiu for dropping out of the group for several months to attend to her newborn grandson, people were quite supportive when another group member had to take a similar-length leave to help her father recover from a stroke.

The Dancing Beauties are not the only group to have these sorts of unspoken rules. In the weeks leading up to a major dance competition, Auntie Wang, the de-facto leader of the Sunset Dance Group, sent the group a very serious WeChat message explicitly stating that the only acceptable reasons for missing practice were medical issues for oneself or for one's parents. Though children and grandchildren were not mentioned in the directive, the implication was understood by all: the demands of the younger generations cannot supersede those of the group. This point was further confirmed when Auntie Wang's pregnant daughter went into labor a month earlier than expected, which prompted Auntie Wang (who missed several days of rehearsals to tend to her daughter and new granddaughter) to send continuous apologetic messages from the hospital maternity ward asking her dance group friends for their understanding.

By the end of my fieldwork, the at-times murky attitudes toward different types of kin relations that shaped the dance groups' strategies to ensure dedication among the members began to coalesce into a clearer picture: participants were duty-bound to tend to their parents and to their spouses in times of need, but extending this same care to one's children and grandchildren was often regarded as a personal choice somewhat different from, or outside of, one's family obligations. Although the traditional moral frameworks of filial piety and family duty apply when dealing with the older generations, these women know very well that their children may never be able to reciprocate these acts of care, and thus they approach the latter relationships with a shrewder, more calculating attitude that provides more space for placing a priority on their own self-interest. But because these internal rules run contrary to the official discourse on family matters, and because they are often left unspoken and unratified by the groups themselves, they require constant—and at times painful—negotiations. The next case is an example of how such negotiations can bring emotionally fraught tensions to the surface, which in turn can test the bonds of both kinship and friendship.

Putting a Price on Care

My next example focuses on a dispute between two Sunset Dance Group women named Wenxie and Liwei. Though they share a close friendship and generally get along well, their different approaches to grandmotherhood are a source of continuous tension. They had apparently been fighting about this for years, but I first learned of their conflicts in the winter of 2016, when Wenxie, Liwei, and I decided to go shopping together after dance practice. There was a seasonal mall on the outskirts of the city that specialized in food and decorations for the upcoming Spring Festival, and our plan was for each of us to go to our respective homes after practice, change clothes, eat lunch, and then meet at a nearby bus station. The holiday was just a few weeks away, and we all wanted to buy snacks and gifts for our families. Liwei and I met at the appointed time and sat down at the bus stop to wait for Wenxie. Five minutes passed. Liwei sent a text message to Wenxie. No response. After another five minutes, Liwei called Wenxie demanding to know her whereabouts. From overhearing Liwei's half of the conversation, I gathered that Wenxie was delayed at home because her three-year-old grandson was eating his lunch very slowly and Wenxie could not leave until the boy had been properly fed. She would be at least another fifteen minutes late. This infuriated Liwei. When she hung up the phone, she immediately turned to me to complain. "The boy has parents!" she began. "Why does she have to feed him when she knows there are people waiting for her?" Liwei has two grandchildren of her own, and she takes pride in the fact that she does not let them interfere with her own social life. For the next ten minutes, Liwei continued to send angry messages to Wenxie telling her to hurry up.

Despite having very little in common on the surface, Liwei and Wenxie are indeed good friends. Whereas Liwei grew up in Chengdu and has educated relatives who are government officials and university professors, Wenxie is from the countryside and moved to Chengdu about ten years earlier to accompany her daughter, a self-made entrepreneur who makes about one million RMB per year.[1] They speak with different accents: Liwei in her standard Chengdu dialect, and Wenxie with a melodic provincial drawl. Liwei prefers long dresses in floral patterns, and she towers above Wenxie, who is less than five feet tall and likes to wear athletic gear. Their different backgrounds are so readily apparent and their friendship so unlikely that they sometimes draw curious looks from strangers. Had they not joined the same dance group, it is unlikely that they would have ever met at all. However, most of the time Liwei and Wenxie did not let their differences get in the way of their friendship, but as this scene at

---

[1] In 2016, one million RMB was equal to approximately 150,000 USD. A person with such an income in Chengdu would be considered very wealthy and would have access to all the luxuries the city had to offer.

the bus stop clearly demonstrated, certain situations could reveal raw disagreements beneath the surface.

When Wenxie finally arrived some thirty minutes after our agreed-upon time, Liwei greeted her by venting her frustrations about having to wait. Wenxie tried to defend herself by explaining that her grandson wanted second helpings and the food had to be reheated. Liwei, however, became even angrier upon hearing this. "Well then his parents could have taken care of him! You could have just gotten up and left and let somebody else feed him more food! Why do you have to be the one to give him seconds? We were waiting for you!" Wenxie offered a placating smile but did not answer. Liwei tried again, this time even more forcefully: "There were other people to take care of your grandson, but we were waiting for you!" Wenxie laughed and shrugged but again she did not answer. She seemed to know that there was nothing she could say to smooth over the differences in outlook she and Liwei had on the subject; while Liwei believed that honoring appointments with friends should take precedence over a toddler's whims, Wenxie placed a priority on her grandchild's needs, even if it meant making her friends wait outside in the cold. I stayed out of it. This was clearly an old disagreement, and neither woman was likely to be moved by the thoughts of a young interloper.

We boarded the bus after a few moments of rather awkward silence. Thankfully, normal conversation resumed well before we reached our destination, and Liwei did not raise the issue again for the rest of the afternoon. We all headed home at the end of the night in good spirits with full shopping bags. I left with the impression that Wenxie simply had more traditional ideas about family obligations than Liwei did. What I did not learn until later was that Wenxie had already taken actions regarding her childcare duties that could not be considered "traditional" by any stretch of the imagination.

Wenxie lives with her son, her son's second wife, and her young grandson. Her son moved to Chengdu soon after his wedding to his first wife in hopes of replicating his sister's phenomenal success. Instead, he found a middling sales job that required frequent travel. Tired of being left to care for their daughter alone, his wife took the child—Wenxie's only grandchild at the time—back to her natal city of Mianyang, located about two hours north of Chengdu. She soon remarried and limited her ties to her ex-husband and to Wenxie, her former mother-in-law. Wenxie's son's second wife is a woman from a rural village in eastern Sichuan, not far from where Wenxie herself was raised. Wenxie disapproved of this relationship from the outset, mostly because she believed her son should not settle for a rural woman now that he had a stable job in the city. However, the woman became pregnant and a wedding was quickly arranged. Wenxie, still stung by the loss of her first grandchild, seemed to have a total change of heart when she learned that she would again have a chance to dote on a baby. She invited her son and her new daughter-in-law to move into her own apartment, which her wealthy daughter had bought for her. After the child—a boy named Wei Wei—was born, Wenxie fed and clothed him from her own modest income of 3,000 RMB (about 450 USD) per month, 2,000 RMB of which was given to her by her daughter as an allowance.

The whole family lived together for a year and a half until Wenxie's daughter-in-law convinced her husband to move their nuclear family into their own apartment. Wenxie was devastated. By both her own and Liwei's accounts, Wenxie was inconsolable that yet another daughter-in-law had denied her the chance to be a doting grandmother. Liwei told me that she used every tactic she could think of to convince Wenxie to stop dwelling on the matter: "I told her, 'if they won't let you take care of the baby, then there's nothing you can do about it. Crying about it certainly won't help.'" Liwei invited Wenxie out for evening walks and told her to try to forget about her family troubles by focusing instead on her own personal life.

After several months of cajoling from Liwei and other members of the Sunset Dance Group, Wenxie finally took this advice to heart and began devoting more of her energy to her own social life. Whereas before she would frequently skip dance practices when her presence was needed at home, she began attending morning practices on a daily basis. Her dancing improved, and she took on additional responsibilities for the group by making WeChat group announcements, collecting dues, and rescheduling rehearsals when the weather prompted cancellations. She began spending more time socializing with Liwei and a few other friends, and she even went on a few overnight sightseeing trips with other dance group members.

Just as Wenxie was beginning to become accustomed to her new life, her son and daughter-in-law suddenly asked to move back in with her. Like many young couples, they were finding it too difficult to work and raise a child at the same time, and they could not afford to pay for daycare; they wanted the round-the-clock childcare that only Wenxie could provide. Against Liwei's and other group members' urgings, Wenxie agreed to let them move back in. ("I told her to never complain to me about them again!" Liwei grumbled as she recounted this story.) Wenxie did, however, surprise her friends by placing new conditions on the living arrangement, requiring her son and daughter-in-law to compensate her for her efforts. She had previously performed all duties related to her grandson's care, including shopping and preparing his meals, but she now demanded monthly payments in exchange for this work.

Wenxie asks for—and receives—300 RMB (about 45 USD) from her son each month, an amount so minimal when compared to the general costs of urban living that it hardly even covers her grandson's room and board, not to mention the fact that live-in nannies who provide the same service cost at least ten times that amount. Moreover, Wenxie confided to me that she does not actually need the money; she doesn't have to save because she knows her daughter will provide for her. Instead, she charges this fee in order to regain a sense of control and dignity over a situation that previously had left her feeling humiliated. "What did they think?" she wondered out loud as we chatted about it after dance practice one day. "That they could just drop me and then pick me back up when it was convenient for them? I won't be taken for granted again."

It is quite unusual for a Chinese grandmother to charge her own son for childcare. There have been some reports of elders suing young couples for a so-called grandchild care fee (*dai sun fei*) in recent years, but such cases are still rare and controversial.[2] Even though exchanging cash, favors, and other valuables among extended family members is a common and indeed foundational feature of Chinese social life (Yang 1994; Yan 1996), putting a price on the everyday acts of caregiving that occur within a domestic unit—much less for one's own grandson—is such an affront to the established norms that Wenxie has only told a few of her closest friends about the arrangement for fear of judgment. For Wenxie, the money served as a simple proxy for a complicated array of impulses. She wanted to convey her pain at having been cast aside, to mete out punishment to her son for mistreating her, and, above all, to make sure that it never happened again. Rather than communicating these fraught emotions directly—an endeavor that offered no guarantee of a satisfactory outcome—Wenxie instead chose to take a symbolic stand that was both easier to ask for and could also serve as a monthly reminder that the terms of the family arrangement were now under her control.

Despite the unorthodox nature of Wenxie's conflict-resolution strategies, scholars have noted elsewhere that blurring the boundaries between care and resources has become commonplace for matters of kinship in the post-reform era. For example, Hong Zhang (2017) has argued that filial piety has been "recalibrated" in order to adhere to post-reform realities, and paying for a nurse for one's ill parent now "counts" as a filial act, even if one is not actually doing the nursing. In Wenxie's case, she was not up to the task of directly asking her son to be more attentive to her feelings. She was, however, able to extract something that counts as more or less the same thing.

Wenxie managed to negotiate an adequate solution by using her ability to provide childcare for her grandson as leverage against her son and daughter-in-law, but it came at the cost of much heartache to all concerned. Her demand for monthly compensation surprised her son, and it especially unsettled her

---

[2] Some high-profile cases of elders successfully suing their children for a *dai sun fei* (grandchild-rearing fee) have appeared on various Chinese news sites since 2014. Most cases seem to involve acrimonious divorces in which one spouse leaves the other and takes the child. The parent of the jilted spouse then sues to recoup the costs of the childcare for the child who has been taken away. See for example http://inews.ifeng.com/yidian/46075914/news.shtml?ch=ref_zbs_ydzx_news, accessed October 28, 2019.

daughter-in-law. In the struggling rural areas where all three of them had grown up, a grandmother would be hard-pressed to attempt such a risky maneuver. This sort of affront to intergenerational solidarity is ill-advised when families must operate as a cohesive unit to survive (Chen, Liu, and Mair 2011; Luo and Zhan 2012; Yan 2016), and rural elders may also lack the social support to act in such an outspoken manner. Wenxie, backed by the financial security offered by her daughter and the social alliances offered by her dance group, successfully came out on top in this intergenerational dispute. Having regained her sense of dignity while also having secured the ability to spend time with her grandson, Wenxie was now eager to avoid further disturbances to her family harmony; she had gone as far as she is willing to go.

Of course, Liwei believes that Wenxie should be willing to go even further in confronting her son and daughter-in-law by refusing to perform certain childcare tasks when these tasks interfere with her personal interests and plans. Liwei's own approach to intergenerational conflict is to maintain the upper hand at all costs, even if it means permanent damage to family ties. Like Wenxie, Liwei's son has two children—a boy and a girl. Also like Wenxie, for a time Liwei's family attempted to live together as three generations, but this arrangement was cut short when her son and daughter-in-law announced that they wanted to get their children away from Liwei's "old-fashioned" child-rearing practices. Liwei was both hurt and furious. Rather than biding her time to find an acceptable outcome like Wenxie did, Liwei instead chose the scorched-earth method: she told her son and daughter-in-law that once they left, they would never again be welcomed back. To this day, Liwei told me, she remains on shaky terms with her son and on even worse terms with her daughter-in-law, but she maintains that she does not care. "I have lots of other things to occupy my time!" she insisted. She is certainly correct in this regard: Liwei is extremely active in the Sunset Dance Group and is seemingly always flitting between one social outing to the next. And as is obvious in how she reacted to Wenxie's plight, Liwei now is also a staunch evangelist for living life on one's own terms.

Confronted with similar challenges, the friends reacted according to their temperaments and priorities. But in both cases, the Sunset Dance Group—or the friendships among the women in the group, to be more precise—played a key role in how the women made their decisions and how they carried out their strategies. For Wenxie, the group provided social support and a diversion when she was feeling abandoned by her son and his wife. It also provided constant pressure to stand up to her son and daughter-in-law and to advocate for her own needs in the form of her friend Liwei, whom she likely would have never met had they not both been members of the same dance group. For Liwei, the group offers constant social connections, many opportunities for recreation, and, ultimately, because the others treat her as something of a leader, it gives her a sense of self-importance.

Wenxie and Liwei have different personalities and different approaches. The same can be said of Teacher Yuan, Qiu, Auntie Yu, and every other retired woman who participates in congregational dance groups. What they have in common is that they are all in the unfamiliar territory of trying to juggle grandmother-hood, friendship, and self-interest at the same time. There is no playbook for maintaining this delicate balance. However, their self-cultivated social groups provide fertile ground for new strategies and norms to grow and circulate.

Looking Ahead

Grandmothers with young children are a ubiquitous sight throughout urban China. In Chengdu, I often saw clusters of middle-aged and elderly women chatting on park benches while toddlers played underfoot and infants napped in strollers. Grandparents lined the sidewalks outside preschools and primary schools in the afternoons, and when hundreds of pairs of little feet finally came streaming out of the gates, the older adults craned their necks anxiously until the children found their way to each of their waiting caregivers. Book bags would soon be transferred onto the elders' backs, and small hands would be gripped firmly by the larger ones before they began the journey home together.

Sweet moments like these are commonplace, but being a grandparent in urban China today can still be a thankless task. As younger generations struggle to balance their high-pressure careers with the demands of childcare, their own parents are often called upon to help ease the domestic burdens on the young couple. Grandparents—and grandmothers in particular—feed, bathe, soothe, and entertain their grandchildren until the little ones are old enough to attend preschool, at which time dropping off and picking up the children may be added to the grandmother's caregiving duties.

Grandparents hoping to take more time for themselves as their grandchildren grow older and more self-sufficient may find these plans thwarted by the revision of the one-child policy (Zhong and Peng 2020). After over thirty years of limiting urban families to one child, a two-child policy was enacted in 2015 to mitigate the effects of population aging and a shrinking labor pool. In a stunning reversal, state-controlled media apparatuses began actively encouraging young couples to have more children. During its decades of enforcement, the one-child policy produced millions of families with a so-called 4-2-1 structure, where four grandparents and two parents dote on a single young child. Stories of grandparents competing for access to their only grandchild abound in popular discourse and neighborhood gossip circles alike. It might make sense, then, for older adults to welcome the prospect of additional grandchildren in the aftermath of the one-child policy's demise. But perhaps not surprisingly, women who spent time cultivating their own interests and social lives feel more ambivalent—or in some cases downright indignant—about the policy shift.

Because I conducted fieldwork from 2014 to 2017, I witnessed some of the initial impacts of the policy change in real time. In general, women in the Dancing Beauties and the Sunset Dance Group were happy that their adult children would have more reproductive choice. A few people shared wistful stories about childhood dreams of large families that were dashed by the one-child policy. Some, like Liwei, welcomed a second grandchild almost immediately after the new law took effect. A few women made their wishes for a second grandchild widely known and bemoaned their adult children's hesitation to expand their families. Most, however, had mixed feelings when confronted with the possibility that their child-rearing years would be extended yet again.

These complicated feelings were often expressed in oblique ways. Auntie Chen, a member of the Dancing Beauties who delighted in teasing me about marriage and children, once asked me point-blank about my plans to become a mother. When I told her that I wanted to wait until I had completed my studies, she replied, "So when you DO have a baby, will your mother take care of it?" I laughed and said that I doubted it: my mother has a very full life of her own, and besides, we don't even live in the same city. Auntie Chen nodded vigorously at this. "Yes, that's exactly right. Your mother is a smart lady!" Auntie Chen had a grandson whom she cared for several days a week. Feeling emboldened by her direct questioning, I decided to be equally blunt in return. "If your daughter has another child," I asked, "will you care for it the way you're taking care of Liang Liang?" She laughed but simply walked away without answering.

In another instance, Auntie Fei (also of the Dancing Beauties) announced at the end of dance practice one day, "I think they are going to try for it. They're going to have another one in the next year or so. "They" referred to Auntie Fei's daughter and son-in-law, who had a four-year-old daughter named Wendy (they gave her an English name to use alongside her Chinese name, a common practice among young middle-class urban couples). "Yes, of course I'm happy," Auntie Fei replied when people congratulated her, "but I hope they don't expect me to take care of another baby."

Auntie Fei was one of the youngest members of the Dancing Beauties and had been retired for only six years when this conversation took place. Most of her retirement had been devoted to caring for Wendy. When her daughter was recovering from childbirth and "sitting the month,"[3] Auntie Fei temporarily

---

[3] "Sitting the month" refers to a set of traditional postpartum practices that are still widely followed in China. Mothers typically stay at home with their infants, avoid work and chores, and are fed nourishing meals to promote healing. These restrictions are meant to protect the health of the mother and newborn.

moved in with her daughter and son-in-law in order to shoulder their household tasks. To allow her daughter to get more rest, Auntie Fei slept in Wendy's room during the first few months and woke with her throughout the night. When her daughter went back to work, Auntie Fei became Wendy's primary caretaker. She arrived at her daughter's apartment each morning shortly after breakfast and did not go home until Wendy was in bed. She even brought Wendy to live with her for weeks at a time so that her daughter and son-in-law could focus on their careers during critical periods. I didn't meet her until after Wendy was old enough to go to preschool, but by Auntie Fei's own account she was so exhausted and stressed that she developed high blood pressure, insomnia, and a persistent pain in her sacrum that still hadn't gone away.

It was no wonder, then, that while Auntie Fei was happy at the prospect of another grandchild, she wasn't eager to repeat the experience of around-the-clock childcare and sleepless nights. Like Qiu, Auntie Fei's social life suffered while she was grandmothering full-time. She skipped most social outings, stopped taking classes at a local old age university (where she had previously been learning ballroom dancing and oil painting), and no longer traveled. When Wendy began preschool at age three, Auntie Fei finally began to go out again. She joked that it felt like retiring for a second time.

During the short but intense conversation in the hallway outside the Dancing Beauties' dance studio, Auntie Fei unloaded a plethora of concerns to her friends. Without her help, it was unlikely that her daughter and son-in-law would be able to manage two children on their own. Auntie Fei didn't want to be the limiting factor to her daughter's family planning, but she also did not feel she could do it again. More crucially, she was eager to keep going out with her friends, cultivating her hobbies, and focusing on herself. "You're so lucky!" Auntie Fei remarked to Jiaming, whose son had already made it clear that he and his wife were content with their one daughter. When Jiaming and another woman from the group suggested that Auntie Fei simply tell her daughter and son-in-law that she would not be available to care for their second child, Auntie Fei resisted the idea. She did not want a confrontation, and she did not want to be embarrassed in case they were not planning to ask for her help. Instead, she chose a strategy of passive avoidance: "I'm just not going to offer. I hope that's enough of a message and they won't ask me about it either."

The last I heard in 2022, Auntie Fei's daughter still had not had a second child. I cannot say for certain whether Auntie Fei eventually made her wishes clear or whether her daughter and son-in-law got the hint from her silence. I also do not know what exactly Auntie Chen meant to convey with her refusal to answer my question about whether she would care for a second grandchild. But what is undeniable is that Chinese women of their generation are not content to place family interests above their own indefinitely. Most young couples are grateful for their parents' efforts, of course, but there are also cases where the grandparents' labor is taken for granted or even—as in Liwei's case—scrutinized and criticized. Chinese media reports and my own observations are filled with stories of elders feeling taken advantage of or being humiliated by this dynamic. As one dance group interlocutor complained, "Sometimes I feel [my daughter and son-in-law] see me as nothing more than a *baomu* [nanny or housekeeper]."

Like their rural counterparts, urban grandmothers have few resources at their disposal to wage a counterinsurgency against the seismic shift in family dynamics. Many—like Qiu and to a certain extent even Wenxie—are afraid that upsetting the younger generation will backfire, and so they do what they can to maintain family harmony. They are all too aware that their children hold most of the cards in any negotiations. This does not mean, however, that urban grandmothers belonging to the sandwich generation must accept China's new inverted family structure at face value. The women in this chapter are all finding new ways of relating to their families that also allow them more space to prioritize their own feelings, needs, and desires. More significantly, they are accomplishing this through conversations with their friends.

The transformation of retirement into a period of personal cultivation has allowed retired women to take the initiative to cultivate and maintain friendships outside of their family circles, and in turn they lean on these friendships to achieve their personal goals. This is not to say that social groups can necessarily function as respites from interpersonal difficulties. Because these friend groups are venues where people can test out emotional intimacies, they are also places where values can clash and conflicts can arise.

Despite these limitations, the social power of friend groups among retired women should not be underestimated. Regular interactions with people in similar circumstances can expose struggling grandmothers to new coping strategies or alternative negotiating tactics when they otherwise would have to suffer in silence. Internal discussions among groups of grandmothers about family dynamics and grandparenting—while seldom arriving at a full consensus—can bring forth new value systems to which the group members feel beholden and accountable.

Of course, although the grandmothers in my examples may have won a few battles, it is far from clear whether they, or any other urban grandparents, will be able to reverse or even stem the trend of the inverted family dynamics that has been taking place for the better part of a century. Such a feat would require social organization and solidarity on a far larger scale than groups of twenty to thirty people can foster. The idea that thousands or even millions of elders will band together to advocate for their collective interests may sound like a grandiose fantasy, but I think it is too soon to completely discount the possibility.

Webpages, blogs, and social media accounts geared toward retirees have proliferated across the Chinese internet in recent years. A brief search for "grandparenting" on any of these platforms yields innumerable results, including blog posts with titles like "I am the child's grandmother, not the nanny!" and think-pieces pondering whether childrearing is the "fate" of all Chinese elders. The comments sections on such posts are usually inundated with additional tales of woe related to caring for grandchildren. Several members of the Sunset Dance Group liked to post links from a site called *laonian hai,* or "old kids," a popular forum that focuses exclusively on issues of interest to older adults. Many of the links contained jokes or funny photos, but occasionally someone would share a poem like the following:

> In the past, there were three ways that a person could fail to be filial
> Now a new type of lacking filial piety has appeared:
> Young people only give birth to children but they do not care for them;
> They put all of the burden of childcare on the backs of the elderly.

While the correlation between opinions expressed on the internet and social reality is admittedly imperfect, the existence of a space devoted to the airing of such complaints demonstrates that the generational solidarity seen in congregational dance groups can be scaled up. These generation-specific internet forums allow tech-savvy elders to learn from one another and offer each other support from afar. They can share the ideas and strategies that originate in their local friend groups with people of their generational cohort throughout the country, and begin to build a collective sense of grievance that can culminate in a sort of collective resistance against a social structure that takes them for granted. It is already clear at this moment that some urban Chinese elders have begun to realize that they can fight back, even if they must fight back with the short end of the stick.

4
Play a Day, Count a Day
● ● ● ● ● ● ● ● ● ● ● ● ● ● ● ● ● ● ● ●

Congregational dance groups are a joy to watch because it seems like the participants are having so much fun. The music is upbeat, the outfits are colorful, and the general atmosphere is lighthearted. Some groups even attract regular audiences at their daily "performances." Throughout my research, people in Chengdu remarked again and again on the dancers' enthusiasm: even those who showed a distaste for the phenomenon grudgingly admitted that it seemed to make the participants happy. Dancers themselves also made frequent reference to their contentment. Many women who participated in congregational dance groups told me that they felt themselves to be fortunate—"幸福." They waxed poetic about their satisfaction with their friendships, their hobbies, and their ability to devote so much time to leisure. "Just look at us," a sixty-seven-year-old dancer declared when I asked for her thoughts on postretirement life. "We are the luckiest generation of Chinese women to have ever lived. No, really! We don't have to work, we are not so poor, and we just have to mind our own mental and physical health. We have such freedom. It's wonderful!"

I only began to hear murmurings of discontent in 2016, when I lived in Chengdu for an extended time and about two years after I initiated the research project. Because the subjects of my interlocutors' complaints were long-standing matters, I credit these late revelations to my interlocutors' increasing trust in me rather than to any changes in external circumstances. The first time anyone expressed serious misgivings about growing older was during an interview with two women I call Auntie Li and Auntie Wu. They were part of a dance group that I met during my preliminary research and then stayed in touch with despite not joining them for regular practices or social gatherings.

In 2016, Auntie Li was fifty-eight years old and Auntie Wu was sixty-five, but both looked about ten years younger than their chronological ages. Auntie Wu was tall, slender, and quite elegant. She always wore well-fitting, color-coordinated outfits and carried a large leather tote bag that seemed to be a bottomless pit of snacks, silk scarves, and extra battery packs for her smartphone. When dancing, she frequently wore oversized sunglasses that made her look a bit like a movie star. Auntie Li also carried an abundance of supplies with her everywhere, but her favored receptacle was a hot pink nylon backpack. While most of the women in their dance group subscribed at least in part to the *dama* aesthetic consisting of short permed hair and bright-colored clothing, Auntie Li truly had a style of her own. She was petite and wiry, and wore her long, graying hair in a braid that reached the small of her back. As she danced, the braid whipped around behind her, giving the distinct impression of a quick-moving cat. She was an avid knitter and seemed to make many of her own clothes, which included things like fringed ponchos, gaucho pants, and woven-leather belts. Auntie Wu and Auntie Li met in the dance group in the mid-2000s and had become good friends by the time I met them. In addition to sharing a favored pastime, they had similar temperaments: they were both sarcastic, observant, and enjoyed making others laugh. In contrast to some of the other women in their group, which consisted of about eighteen women who mostly lived in the neighborhoods directly abutting the small park where they danced, both Auntie Li and Auntie Wu paid attention to current events, particularly at the local level. Occasionally, they would in the course of conversation reference local news stories like the groundbreaking of a new shopping mall or a local official accused of taking bribes. But until the interview in question, the two of them had been consistently jovial and upbeat in all of our interactions.

The interview took place after a weekday dance practice in the park. My initial intention was to ask Auntie Li about what it was like to transition out of the workforce, but Auntie Wu joined us when she saw us sitting in a covered pagoda before the interview began. The conversation began uneventfully with some small talk about the women's families, but the tone of the conversation palpably shifted when I asked them for their thoughts on the general plight of Chinese elders. Auntie Li's voice was tense as she began: "Things look good if you are doing a shallow observation. But if you were to come back in twenty years, you would see a disaster. Come back when we are in our seventies and eighties and our kids are in their fifties. It will be a disaster." As she made this ominous prophesy, Auntie Wu sat beside her and nodded along in agreement.

Auntie Li and Auntie Wu spent the next thirty minutes taking turns to elaborate. Health insurance is inadequate, and most people are one serious illness away from financial trouble, Auntie Wu explained. Auntie Li added that adult children—most of them singletons due to the one-child policy—cannot be relied on for eldercare because they are struggling to make ends meet for their own families. Both women spoke at length about the inadequacy of institutional eldercare options: "The nice ones are very luxurious," Auntie Li told me, "but on 2,000 RMB a month [pension] they won't take you! The kind that we *can* afford are terrible. I've gone to see them. They don't take care of you at those places. They put a bunch of rickety beds in a run-down building, and drape a raggedy blanket on each bed. That's what you can get for 1,000–2,000 yuan. We couldn't suffer those conditions!" Auntie Wu vigorously agreed: "Of course it's different for those with money, but most people don't have money."

They shared a long list of grievances during our conversation. Among the subjects they covered were the one-child policy, corruption and graft, condescending and ineffective policies, the exorbitant cost of medical treatment, and the even more dire circumstances of people who do not own an apartment. They raged about the failures of the central government, the municipal government, and the local government. "So you want to study old people?" Auntie Li challenged me at one point in the conversation. "No one can find solutions for old people's problems." Why, I asked, did they spend so much time dancing? If the future was so bleak, then why did they enjoy themselves so much? Auntie Wu chuckled in response.

"Yes, we dance. We dance and we're happy. They say that if you don't dance and if you don't play mahjong then you'll start paying attention to politics." Here, the two of them broke out into a hearty laugh. "So they keep us dancing and playing! And we are happy when we dance. Foreigners must come here and think, 'Chinese people are so happy—they dance and play mahjong all day!' What they don't know is that our hearts are actually full of bitterness."

I was stunned by these revelations. Again, this conversation marked the first time I had heard a *dama* present anything other than a generally rosy picture of her life. I asked them how they dealt with the psychological burden of knowing that such potentially difficult times were ahead. "I just don't think about it!" Auntie Li answered laughing. "At least for now we have our porridge money." In the Sichuanese vernacular, having "porridge money," or 稀饭钱, means being able to pay for the bare necessities of life but nothing more. "Why would I waste time thinking about it?" she continued. "There's nothing I can do about it. I don't have money to buy better insurance. I can't have more children. There's nothing I can do to make my future more secure. There's nothing I can do."

Perhaps seeing the pained look on my face, Auntie Wu stepped in to offer her outlook. "It's like this," she explained. "For us, it's just one day at a time: we play a day, live a day. Play a year, live a year. We keep our attention on the present." She used the Sichuanese word for play—*shua*. Auntie Li solemnly agreed. "Yes, *shua yi tian, suan yi tian* [play a day, count a day]. We enjoy ourselves while we can. When you get old what you need to do is let go of any hope you had for the future."

The Sichuanese dialect is full of colorful terms and expressions that carry multilayered meanings, of which *shua* is a prime example. On the simplest level, it means "to play." A mother might send her child outside to *shua*, or someone might be described to be *shua*-ing a video game. It can also mean engaging in leisure, entertainment, or travel activities: one could say that one plans to spend a day at the mall to *shua* or ask someone where they are going to *shua* on their upcoming vacation. Finally, it can mean dissipation or decadence. To say that a child likes to *shua* is also to say she is not studious. To say that a young adult spends her time engaging in *shua* is also to say that she is immature or unfocused. In each case, the word calls to mind a carefree, unserious, and idle attitude. I was puzzled about how women with so many serious cares could give the word such a central place in describing their lives.

In the months and years following my interview with Auntie Li and Auntie Wu, I heard numerous other accounts that contained echoes of this conversation. Several people repeated what Auntie Li said nearly verbatim—that they have no hopes for the future and only focus on finding enjoyment in the present moment. I also continued to hear people say that they felt tremendously fortunate. Sometimes the same person offered these opposing points of view on separate occasions. The enjoyment and the bitterness seemed to be two halves of the same whole, or two ends of a seesaw that continuously teeters back and forth. But both types of comments came up rarely, even with my prompting: for the most part, the *dama* who participate in dance groups possess a dogged determination to focus on what is going on right in front of them. Moments of reflection on the past or anticipation of the future were as fleeting as they were uncommon among the members of both dance groups I spent time with. While some might characterize this trait as shallowness or lack of self-awareness—the derisive dimensions of the *dama* stereotype certainly carry these undertones—I contend that it is an intentional strategy for living well within the constraints of their circumstances.

People adopting a blasé attitude about the future in the face of uncertainty is not unique to China. What is interesting about the Chinese case, however, is that these attitudes cut across socioeconomic classes and reflect generational experiences rather than financial insecurity. The retired women I encountered in Chengdu had varying degrees of wealth as well as different ways of handling uncertainty. The common threads that tied their stories together was their investment of time and resources in leisure.

"Now They Have Done Nothing"

In early summer 2017, one of my interlocutors from the Dancing Beauties posted an internet meme in the group's WeChat forum. It was a photo of four *People's Daily* newspapers stacked one on top of another so that only the headlines were visible. Together, the headlines and their accompanying dates—circled in red—told the story of China's rapidly evolving state-society relations with succinct and almost poetic clarity:

1985: Having one child is good; the state will provide eldercare
1995: Having one child is good; the state will help provide eldercare
2005: Do not rely on the state for eldercare
2012: Delaying retirement is good; provide your own eldercare

I discovered very early on in my fieldwork that I would not be able to carry out research on congregational dancers without WeChat. Resolutely defying the conventional wisdom about retirees' aversions to the internet and social media, my interlocutors spent an incredible amount of time attending to WeChat—hanging out in large group chats with each other, taking and posting photos, and scrolling through friends' posts to find photos to "like." When I finally downloaded the app and joined the group chats, I ended up quickly shutting off notifications and message alerts on my phone because it turned out that the women sent hundreds of messages a day to each other. Each morning began with a series of greetings. These would most frequently be in the form of emoticons and gifs, but occasionally a hand-typed message wishing others a good morning would also appear. The barrage of messages would continue at a steady pace throughout the day and would slacken only during the periods of time during which the women were in each other's physical presence, such as during dance practices or social activities. Each day concluded with another slew of messages in the late evening wishing each other a peaceful night or sweet dreams.

All this is to say that sending funny photos and other viral internet content is common practice in the dancers' WeChat groups. Most of the time, however, everyone allows these posts to pass by without comment; long stretches of chat transcripts entail nothing more than continuous non sequiturs. For example, directly before the eldercare meme appeared, someone had posted an article about foods to avoid in hot weather, which was followed by a video of a golden retriever wearing overalls, to which someone else responded with a gif of Vladimir Putin waving to a pigeon. The newspaper headline meme elicited a different reaction. Within minutes of its appearance, several people chimed in with snarky one-liners and laughing face emojis. Several others added slightly more serious commentary: "They really fooled us!" wrote Jun, who was laid off in 1999, one year after her husband initiated a divorce so that he could pursue a younger woman. "Delay retirement? As if anyone had a choice!" wrote Ruiqing, who was laid off from her job in 2002 and now works part-time as an accountant for an auto repairs company. The group sustained this discussion for over thirty minutes before the chat resumed its usual rhythm of silly gifs, web links, and posed photos. No one in the group ever mentioned the meme or its contents again.

However fleeting, the meme had clearly managed to touch a nerve. By virtue of their ages, the women who participate in dance groups have endured some of the brunt of China's dramatic social changes. Again, most of them belong to China's baby-boom generation, born in the years between 1949 and 1965. Many came of age during the Cultural Revolution and never completed their formal educations. They were assigned jobs in state-owned enterprises or other urban work units upon completing vocational training but faced layoffs and forced retirements when the state privatized or reformed SOE's in the late 1990s and 2000s. When they were young, the state made a promise to take care of urban workers from the cradle to the grave, only to renege on that promise in order to make the Chinese economy more competitive. Though general quality of life has dramatically improved as a result of these reforms, it is difficult to overstate the sense of precariousness that living through these changes has imparted on this generation of people. These women are now in their fifties to seventies, their children are grown, and they are facing old age in circumstances radically different from what they anticipated when they were younger.

A few days after the initial appearance of the *People's Daily* meme in the Dancing Beauties' WeChat group, the image appeared again in my own WeChat inbox accompanied by a note: "We should talk about this when you come over later." The message was from a woman I call Auntie Yang. She was a friend of one of my mother's friends, and I met her at a social gathering years earlier during a family visit to Chengdu. I reached out to her when I began my fieldwork, and we occasionally chatted about her participation in an all-female choir group. In truth, I kept up my visits to Auntie Yang because she was so kind and always made me feel welcome. She was a talented cook who experimented with traditional Chinese medicinal ingredients, and her home always smelled wonderfully of spices and herbs. She lived on the first floor of a highrise building in a quiet residential development. The apartment itself was quite modest, but it had its own large backyard—an extremely rare luxury in urban China—in which she and her husband grew their own vegetables, cultivated flowers, and even kept a koi pond. Though I arrived each time with the intention of asking her questions relevant to my research, we often simply spent a few hours looking over her most recent vacation photos or touring her garden. I had been looking forward to visiting her for weeks when I received her WeChat message.

When I arrived that afternoon, Auntie Yang wasted no time before getting to the point. The meme had evidently spread like wildfire through various retiree interest groups on WeChat. While she served tea and fruit on her spacious patio overlooking the garden, Auntie Yang told me that the image had been circulated among her friends in both her choir group and her prayer group (she converted to Christianity shortly after retiring), and from what she described, it sounded like it had caused as much of a commotion in those group chats as it had in the Dancing Beauties' group. Auntie Yang explained that the meme had resonated with her deeply. "They told us that they would take care of it," she said, in a voice layered with anger and defiance. "That's why they told us all to have one child. And now that we're actually old they're backing down from their promises. They can't take care of us, we've got to take care of ourselves [靠自己]." "If we're lucky enough to have friends," she concluded, "maybe we can take care of each other [互相靠]."

Auntie Yang has one adult son who was born in 1985, six years after the one-child policy was implemented. He displayed tremendous athletic abilities as a child, so she and her husband poured all their resources into cultivating his talents. Their efforts seemed to pay off when he was signed by a team in Europe and moved abroad, but then he aged out of the sport and returned to China with no college education and unpromising job prospects. He eventually found work as a children's coach at a school near the city center. He went on to marry a woman with a stable if not lucrative career, and the couple now lives with the wife's parents, who take care of their toddler son while they work long hours. Auntie Yang is not disappointed in how her son turned out. He is hard working and kind, and he visits whenever he can. In an ideal world, she would spend more time with him and her grandchild but understands that he cannot be in two places at once. Instead, her resentment is reserved for the state—or as she calls it—"them." When I asked her whether she thought the newspaper headlines were real or rather photo-shopped by someone hoping to make a point, she waved her hand impatiently in front of my face and told me that it did not matter: regardless of its provenance, the image captured an essential truth about her personal experience of the past forty years. "We were the generation that got the worst of it," she said. "When we were young, they demanded so many sacrifices from us, and in return they promised us that they would educate our children, make sure we have jobs, and then take care of us when we are old. Now they have done nothing."

"Nothing" is a bit of an exaggeration in this case. Auntie Yang and her husband both have generous pensions from their former public-sector jobs. They own their home and have above-average health-care plans as part of their pension packages. They take at least two domestic vacations per year—sometimes flying but more often taking road trips to scenic areas in their SUV along with a few other retired couples in a caravan. At the time of this interview, they were also in the midst of planning a multi-country European sightseeing trip with a small group of friends. When I tried to point this out, Auntie Yang cackled out loud and explained that the only way they can afford the trips is because one of their travel buddies is a part owner of a tour company and can get them special deals. In other words, Auntie Yang is playing with more than just "porridge money."

In light of her relative financial comfort, Auntie Yang's discontent may be somewhat of a puzzle. By all measures, she has much to be grateful for and very little to complain about. And yet she shares the "bitterness" mentioned by Auntie Wu and Auntie Li. To understand why Auntie Yang is unhappy with her situation despite having many resources at her disposal, one needs to simply return to the *People's Daily* newspaper meme. The key here is how each policy change is presented as a matter of fact and without reference to earlier realities. When it comes to the business of aging, Auntie Yang and her husband—along with millions of others—did not know that they were on their own until the ground had already shifted underneath them. In its relentless pursuit of modernity and development over the past few decades, the state has implemented numerous whiplash-inducing policies that have left this generation of people scrambling to come up with ways to take care of themselves. Auntie Yang has focused her ire on the one-child policy, which forced her to put all her eggs in one basket, so to speak, and invest heavily in one son who may not be able to repay her in the form of eldercare due to the many competing claims on his time and money. But the adverse effects of this policy were unquestionably exacerbated by the economic reforms that broke the state's earlier promise to take care of urban residents from the cradle to the grave. All this is to say that Auntie Yang's perspectives about growing older are as much (if not more) influenced by her experiences as they are by her purchasing power. Her anger stems from a sense of having been betrayed or abandoned.

The result is that even someone with enviable personal resources like Auntie Yang still must find her own way to make up for the care that the state promised her in exchange for her reproductive sacrifices. Having made these sacrifices to no avail, she must find other sources of support since she also cannot rely on her only son. I brought the conversation back to eldercare and asked Auntie Yang what she plans to do now that the state can no longer be relied upon. Had she visited any eldercare facilities? Could she imagine herself living in one? She sidestepped the questions in her response. She told me that she and her husband intend to co-invest in a large property outside the city with several longtime friends and move there when they get older. The idea is that they will keep each other company and take care of each other as they physically decline. It turns out that this is what she meant when she said that she and her friends would rely on each other as they grow older.

I cannot say whether Auntie Yang's plans for eldercare will pan out or if it is a pipe dream. Auntie Yang does not seem to know either. I brought it up a few more times over the remaining months that I was in Chengdu, and each time Auntie Yang was happy to talk about it but declined to go into specifics about where the property might be, whether she envisioned hiring any staff, or how the costs might be split among the friends. Instead, she focused on how they would spend their days: "We can play mahjong in the afternoons," she once said. "We can sing karaoke; we can do whatever we want." She did not say it in so many words, but her emotional investment in the idea of growing older with her friends grew out of a desire to build a vision for the future independent of official institutions, which she has deemed unreliable. At least for now, Auntie Yang has decided that her best bet is to continue cultivating her friendships in the hope that these bonds will pay off in the future.

Counting the Days

Most of my interlocutors approached the subject of eldercare and their own aging from indirect angles. After the eye-opening interview with Aunties Li and Wu, I began asking the women in my dance groups about their thoughts or plans on eldercare with some regularity. Some of these forays were answered with platitudes about not wishing to be a burden on their children, some were met with vague murmurs of dread or resignation, and some were brushed off altogether. However, as time went on, I noticed that most of my interlocutors did wish to talk about their anxieties, albeit in oblique ways——most readily offering their feelings while expressing sympathy for the plight of others.

One such conversation occurred when a woman from the Sunset Dance Group whom I call Auntie Liu offered to walk to my grandmother's house with me after dance practice. Auntie Liu was one of the founding members of the Sunset Dance Group who, along with six or seven other women from her neighborhood, began meeting in the mornings to dance when they were all laid off from their jobs in 2003. At the time, they were in their mid- to late forties. By the time I met her in 2016, Auntie Liu had perfected the routines of what she called her *tuixiu shenghuo*, or retiree life. She told me that she began her days with the Sunset Dance Group in the park, then headed home to make lunch, sometimes stopping at the market along the way. After lunch and a nap, she and her husband (who retired in 2013) liked to read together on their walled-in porch. She enjoyed online serialized fiction about ancient China, while he preferred to research travel destinations. A lot of the time, she admitted with a laugh, they both ended up playing games on their smartphones instead. Her husband then did household chores while she cooked dinner, which they ate in front of the television. She always took an after-dinner walk ("it helps with my digestion") and sometimes convinced her husband to do the same ("he would sit in the house all day if I let him!").

Auntie Liu happened to live just around the corner from my grandmother, and we frequently shared walks when I was heading in that direction after dance practice. We would spend the twenty minutes or so chatting while she walked her bicycle alongside. On this particular morning, she was distraught over a scene she had witnessed the previous weekend. She had been out on one of her evening walks in the neighborhood, she told me, when she saw an older man collapse on the sidewalk. The man was conscious and speaking, but his wife was struggling to get him back onto his feet, so Auntie Liu rushed over to see if she could help. When she drew nearer, she was shocked to recognize the couple as Mr. Jiang and Ms. Wang, the parents of her son's childhood friend. The two families had frequently spent time together when their sons were children but had fallen out of touch. Auntie Liu poignantly took time to describe the relieved look on Ms. Wang's face when she recognized Auntie Liu. With the help of a few passersby, they eventually managed to bring Mr. Jiang to the hospital in a taxi, where doctors discovered that he had suffered a stroke. Auntie Liu recalled each of the harrowing events—the collapse, the attempts to revive, the hailing of the taxi, watching Mr. Jiang be admitted to the hospital, and receiving Ms. Wang's call with news about the stroke a few hours later—in breathless detail. Throughout the account, she repeatedly interrupted herself to exclaim, "This was such a tragedy!"

Over the next months, Auntie Liu and I walked together after dance practice about a dozen more times, and each time she would tell me more about Mr. Jiang and Ms. Wang. Their son (their only child), she revealed, had emigrated to the United States to work in the software industry. He still had not received a green card so could not return to China to visit his parents without jeopardizing his work visa. Mr. Jiang and Ms. Wang had considered trying to move to the United States as well, but decided against it when they realized they would be isolated and bored, especially since their son was single and had no children for them to look after. They had been doing all right until the stroke. Each of them spent time on their hobbies—she on a choir group and he on online Chinese chess—and took a nightly walk together for exercise. But Mr. Jiang's stroke proved to be devastating for their quality of life: despite surviving, he needed months of rehabilitative care to regain mobility. Things took an even worse turn when, about six weeks after Mr. Jiang was admitted to the hospital, Ms. Wang was also hospitalized for a preexisting medical problem that was exacerbated by the stress of caring for her husband. Mr. Jiang had since been moved to a rehabilitative center in another neighborhood, while Ms. Wang was in the internal medicine ward at the local hospital; the couple had no way to visit one another. In each of our conversations, Auntie Liu bitterly bemoaned the situation and its lack of recourse while I commiserated. She often wondered aloud, "Without their child here, what can they possibly do? How can they get better?"

The subtext to Auntie Liu's anxieties for her friends was that her own son also lived in the United States. He had attended a graduate program at the University of Texas, where he met and married a fellow student from China. He and his wife got good jobs after graduation and are raising their two young children in the Austin area. Auntie Liu and her husband have visited Texas several times but have made no bid to join their son there permanently. Life is boring in America, Auntie Liu explained, repeating the phrase that I have often heard from recent immigrants from China to the United States when describing what living in America feels like: *hao shan, hao shui, hao wuliao* [great mountains, great water, great boredom]. She would have to give up the dance group, there was nothing interesting within walking distance of their son's suburban home, and she and her husband cannot even understand the shows on TV. "There's nothing worse for one's health than that kind of isolation," she said, and I could not help but agree. Over time, Auntie Liu revealed additional reasons for their hesitation. They did not know if they would get approved for longer-term visas or green cards (some of their acquaintances in similar situations had been denied). They got along with their son and daughter-in-law during their visits, but were not sure if they could live together harmoniously long-term. Most of all, their son had never explicitly asked them to move in with him.

Auntie Liu never said that she wished her son would ask. She never voiced a desire for him to move back to China, either. She was proud of him and told anyone who would listen about his successful, comfortable life in Austin. In fact, she was one of the first women I became closer to in the Sunset Dance Group because she enjoyed chatting about America with someone else who had been there. However, she extended none of this same grace to Mr. Jiang and Ms. Wu's son, at whose feet she laid much of the blame for his parents' untenable situation. If only he had settled down in China, she lamented on multiple occasions, his parents would not be in such a conundrum. She lambasted him for his bachelor lifestyle. "His house is not a home," she told me, relaying information from Ms. Wang, with whom she had renewed a friendship since their fateful encounter on the sidewalk. "He lives in a small apartment. The only thing he knows how to cook is a whole chicken inside a giant pot of rice. He cooks it on Sunday and then eats it all week, even after it has started to smell funny. That's not the kind of environment for older people." If he lived his life in such a way that better accommodated his parents, she mused, they would have more incentive to move to the United States and be cared for by him in their old age.

I do not think that the irony of her criticizing Mr. Jiang and Ms. Wang's son while praising her own was lost on Auntie Liu. Though she never said so directly, Mr. Jiang and Ms. Wang's misfortunes preoccupied her so much because the same thing could easily happen to her and her husband. At one point, Auntie Liu sighed in a resigned manner and said, "There's nothing to do for us old people here but to help each other when we can. We can't rely on our children anymore."

While I have previously written about dance and the enjoyment of hobbies as acts of self-determination, it is clear from what Auntie Liu says here that voluntary group associations among urban retirees are also taken up as a means of self-preservation. With the state safety networks eroding while traditional practices of in-home eldercare becoming more difficult to attain for Chinese families, older adults must find alternative means of social support. Auntie Liu could not give me hard numbers, but she insisted that "very many" of her peers were in the same situation as herself and of the unlucky couple whose plight she anxiously followed. On paper, these retirees are among the most privileged in China: their children are living abroad or in larger cities because they have well-paying or prestigious jobs. Because they were the first generation of parents to be limited to just one child, people like Auntie Liu often worked hard to give their children every possible advantage. Their children's successful careers, then, are the long hoped-for result of years of anxiety and sacrifice.

But in the process of evaluating her life while standing on the cusp of old age, it was clear that Auntie Liu viewed her son's accomplishments as a sort of Pyrrhic victory. Successful adult children's accomplishments also work to strain family ties because they prevent the children from providing care or companionship for their parents. Still, Auntie Liu counts herself as lucky. Because her son is married and has two children, she has a clear role in their family and feels useful and wanted when she is with them. "At least I can be a grandmother when I am in Texas," Auntie Liu once explained. "I can't help my son with his career like I might have been able to if he had stayed in China, but at least I can help watch his kids." In other words, her grandmother role offers her an anchor in an otherwise wholly disorienting view of the future. Others, like her friends Mr. Jiang and Ms. Wang, do not have even this meager asset.

And yet in the weeks and months after her friends' crisis unfolded, Auntie Liu did not devote more energy toward cultivating closer ties with her son and grandchildren. Over the years that I knew her, she mentioned several times that she preferred to take her son's lead on the terms of their relationship. She never pushed for more visits or calls, and only occasionally sent her son messages over WeChat. None of this changed despite the anxiety that being witness to Mr. Jiang and Ms. Wang's troubles obviously gave her. Instead, Auntie Liu kept at her "retiree life." The doubt and turmoil that had consumed her for months did not push her to deviate from her habits, which she had cultivated over many years to maximize relaxation and leisure.

The last time I saw Auntie Liu was when I was returning to the United States at the end of my fieldwork in 2017 and improbably ran into her at in the terminal at the Los Angeles International Airport. She and her husband were on their way to Austin for their annual visit. We only realized that we had been on the same flight when we disembarked. We happily chatted as we walked down the long corridors toward the Department of Homeland Security checkpoint, taking multiple photos along the way to post to the Sunset Dance WeChat group. When we reached the checkpoint and had to part ways because there were separate lines for domestic and foreign nationals, I made a joke that perhaps in the future she would receive American citizenship and we could stand in the same line together. "Oh no," she replied. "I couldn't give up my fun that easily. Next time you see me, I'll be dancing in the park as always."

All the retired women mentioned thus far harbor varying degrees of recognition that their present conundrums vis-à-vis their futures in general and eldercare in particular can be traced to government policies. Aunties Li, Wu, and Yang all explicitly blame the state for breaking promises and leaving older adults with a bad bargain. While Auntie Li and Auntie Wu characterize their participation in congregational dancing and other leisure activities as the only consolation they have in an otherwise bleak landscape, Auntie Yang frames her group activities with other retirees as ways to mitigate some of the risk of growing older without a safety net.

There are others, however, who turned toward *shua* in response to an acute crisis. The most prominent example of this that I saw was with Dancing Beauties member Ying. Her eighty-nine-year-old mother slipped on the stairs and strained her shoulder while trying to break her fall with her arm. At the hospital, she had the misfortune of encountering a young doctor who, without first taking an X-ray, assumed that the shoulder was dislocated and pulled on her arm as hard as he could until it fractured. What began as a simple injury became an extended stay at an osteopathic hospital. Meanwhile, Ying's ninety-year-old father, Mr. Wei, was completely helpless in his wife's absence because he had never learned to cook or keep house. Ying's older brother began going to Mr. Wei's house each evening to prepare meals. One night, he was delayed by work and Mr. Wei was very hungry by the time he arrived. In his desire to speed up the cooking process, Mr. Wei bent down to retrieve a clove of garlic from a bottom cabinet, lost his balance, and fell. His son helped him into bed and called a doctor, who determined that Mr. Wei had sprained his back. What was already a difficult situation thus devolved into a domestic catastrophe: Ying's mother was hospitalized while her father was simultaneously bed-bound. Both elders needed their meals delivered, their clothes laundered, and their bodies bathed. Even though this caregiving work was spread among three siblings, Ying became so overwhelmed that she stopped attending dance practices.

I saw her just twice during this period of crisis—once when she stopped by dance practice to say hello on her way to buy groceries, the other when she joined the group for a lunch outing at a buffet restaurant on a rare afternoon off. Both times, Ying blithely joked that her parents should have worked out a more convenient schedule for their respective falls because it was thoughtless of them to be bedridden at the same time. She longed to be back at the dance group. She often sent dozens of messages into the group WeChat while keeping her parents company at their bedsides. While she graciously accepted the other women's sympathy and well-wishes, her own contributions to the group chat were composed primarily of dance videos, funny gifs, and nature photography. She seldom volunteered information about her parents, and only responded to queries with one-line replies. It was difficult to get a sense of her mental or emotional state during this time.

Both of Ying's parents eventually recovered from their injuries, though they never regained their full independence. They were both more cautious and frail. Ying and her siblings took over many aspects of their activities of daily living, including grocery shopping and errands. When she returned to regular practices about six weeks after her mother's fall, something about Ying was noticeably different. She had always been quick-witted and quick to laugh, but her humor became downright sardonic at times. During one of our brief encounters while her parents needed full-time care, Ying vowed that she and her husband would move to an eldercare facility when they got older. That way, she said, they would not be a burden on their son in the same way that her parents were currently a burden to her. She listed the benefits of living in an eldercare facility: they have daily organized activities, everyone is similar in age and life experience so you always have someone to talk to, if you are too tired to cook you can just to go the canteen. She sounded a bit like she was trying to convince herself that this would not be such a bad way to live. Her optimism was resolute, if somewhat forced.

About a month after she returned to dance practices, Ying said something that made me realize her outlook on the future had shifted. During a post- practice excursion to a nearby Carrefour market with a few other women, she began to complain about her son: he does not see how tired she is, he does not care how much she has sacrificed for him, he would not be able to reciprocate the care that he received from her. "He will never do what I do for my parents now," she exclaimed as the others in the group sympathized. "You're right," someone else chimed in. "What will happen to us when we're that old?" Ying answered with her usual jovial tone, *"ba women tai chuqu shuaile."*—they'll carry us out and throw us away.

The experience of caring for her elderly parents day in and day out was clarifying for Ying, perhaps because the exhaustion of the caregiving made her realize that her son would not be capable of enduring the same. Whatever the reason, Ying responded to her parents' health crises and gradual decline by taking every opportunity to enjoy herself. She began to travel as frequently as once a month. Most of her trips were to relatively nearby places like Ya'an, a city south of Chengdu known for its mild climate, and Kunming, the capital of Yunnan Province. However, she also applied for a passport and traveled to Hong Kong, then Thailand, then Malaysia. Each time, she went with tour groups geared toward retirees. In between these travels, Ying performed her filial duties to her parents diligently and without complaint. She gave no indication that she resented them, but her attitude toward the rest of her life was noticeably different.

Unlike Aunties Li, Wu, and Yang, all of whom took historical views of their current predicaments and blamed state policies, both Auntie Liu and Auntie Ying have more personal grievances and worries about growing older. It comes down to a matter of interest and personality: Ying was never one to pay much attention to the news or politics, so it was in keeping with her usual habits that she perceived this experience through the lens of her daily life. Auntie Liu, similarly, preferred to steer clear of political topics; she once told me that she made a point to leave the room whenever her husband turned on the nightly state news broadcast.

After I returned to the United States in late 2017, I continued to stay abreast of Ying's travels through her WeChat posts. In autumn 2018 I saw that she and her husband had traveled to Dunhuang, an ancient Silk Road outpost and famous tourist spot in northwestern Gansu Province. She looked resplendent in her colorful dresses, posing in front of grottos and sand dunes. By the time I saw the album, it had already garnered dozens of compliments from fellow *dama*. I added a comment to the long list admirers: "Ying, you look so wonderful!," I wrote. She replied to all of us with a gracious, humble post interspersed with emojis: "Thank you to all my sisters for your kind comments. Your friendship and support have touched my heart. May we all have exciting adventures. We need to make the most of the time we have. Play a day, count a day!"

New Realities, New Expectations

Retired women in China today are acutely aware of the echoes of history that continue to affect their lives in untold ways, almost as acutely as they are aware of their own impending old age and mortality. There was a palpable sense—percolating just beneath the surface—that the good days were numbered. But many of these women choose to redouble their focus on finding joy in the daily routines of texting friends, dancing, cooking, caring for grandchildren, and socializing rather than try to forestall a potentially bleak old age. The past events that set them on this trajectory cannot be undone, so why bother with such bitter thoughts more often than is necessary?

And yet, as the interview with Auntie Wu and Auntie Li demonstrates, there are moments when the feelings of resentment and fear that are normally kept at bay do not comply with one's efforts to contain them to the margins. This chapter was about these moments—the events and triggers that bring them to the fore, how they unfold, and how they are assimilated into the worldview that the *dama* make for themselves and each other. More significantly, it was also about the ways in which these moments are meaningfully de-centered in these women's lives through jokes, irony, and the focus on leisurely activities that fall under the catch-all *shua*.

The women featured in this chapter are hardly the only people who are concerned about what growing old in China in the coming decades will look like. A sense of abandonment drives a significant portion of the narrative about aging in China today. But despite what the earlier *People's Daily* meme might suggest, the evidence indicates that the central government is, in fact, actively trying to find solutions. I conducted a survey of instances of the term "养老," or "eldercare," in *People's Daily* newspaper archives from 1947 to 2017, and found that attention to this issue has dramatically increased over the past several decades.

The most high-profile solution that government organizations have offered is to promote the Confucian ethic of filial piety in order to guilt families into taking care of their own elders. Posters, commercials, and public service announcements promoting filial piety have also sprung up in Chinese cities in recent years. I saw them daily in Chengdu, where they would appear on buildings, fencing, and at bus stops. In 2013 the state even passed a "filial piety" law that made it illegal for adult children to neglect their elderly parents. The law is vague—children are required to visit their parents "often" and "occasionally" send greetings, which makes it difficult to enforce. However, those found in violation of it may be put on a credit blacklist that makes getting a loan or a library card impossible, and unhappy elders can now even sue their un-filial children under this law. Given how deeply filial piety runs in Chinese culture, it should not be surprising that the state has once again turned to promoting so-called family values as a means of getting people out of the bind that the state itself put them in. Filial piety has been customary throughout China for at least two thousand years. For centuries, Chinese elders could reasonably expect to grow old at home with sons and daughters-in-law as their primary caretakers. But times have clearly changed.

In a heartbreaking case that perfectly captures how kinship ideologies on the aging process collide with new post-reform realities, in the winter of 2017 a widower in his eighties named Mr. Han placed himself up for adoption. One of his sons had immigrated to Canada about fifteen years earlier, and he was estranged from his other son. Mr. Han told his neighbors that he was terrified of dying alone. Feeling like he had no recourse, he posted the adoption ad at a busy bus stop. It read, "Searching for a caring family to adopt me until my death." Unfortunately, Mr. Han indeed died alone, in May 2018 His neighbors found his body a few days after he had died, and his heart-wrenching story soon went viral on the Chinese internet. Online commentators were quick to blame his sons. "The two sons do not support their father because of their modern education," one wrote. "China's five thousand years of tradition has been ruined

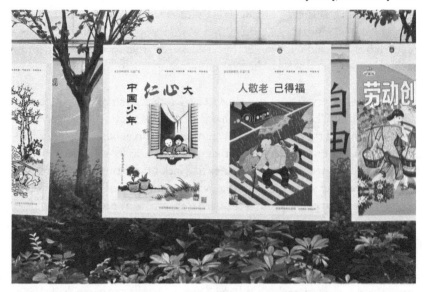

FIGURE 6 Posters promoting "Chinese cultural values," including filial piety, hanging on a line in a Chengdu neighborhood. (Photo by Claudia Huang)

by modern times" ("Elder in His 80s Pastes 'Plea for Adoption' on Street Corner," n.d.).

This may be an understandable conclusion to draw, but the evidence does not support it. In fact, scholarly research has found that filial piety is not necessarily declining. Sociologist Becky Hsu's three-year project on Chinese definitions of happiness found that young people frequently refer to their ability (or lack thereof) to perform their filial duties to their parents as a primary metric of personal happiness (Hsu and Madsen 2019). Furthermore, Hong Zhang (2017) has argued that filial piety itself has been redefined to suit post-reform realities—for example, hiring a caretaker for your parents is now considered a filial act, even if you yourself cannot do the caring. In other words, if people are truly unable to take care of their elderly parents, it is unlikely due to the younger generation's weak moral fiber or lack of respect for Chinese cultural traditions. Instead, filial duties are neglected because circumstances render such acts of care financially or geographically impossible. In any case, and as much as the state may wish otherwise, the bonds of kinship are no longer sufficient for providing the care that Chinese elders will need in the coming years.

Another idea that has received substantial attention and investment focuses on recruiting younger retirees to take care of older, more dependent ones. The idea is that people who volunteer as caretakers now—still-limber retirees in their sixties or perhaps late fifties—will receive care from a new group of volunteers later, when they reach their eighties or nineties. Called the Mutual

Support Model, this type of caregiving setup was borrowed from a similar "time-banking" mutual care system that was developed in Japan in the early 1990s. It has achieved some success in rural villages, where people tend to know each other well, and where the care often occurs within preexisting social networks.

The cities, however, are a different story: I interviewed municipal government officials in Chengdu as well as managers of a domestic elder engagement organization, and they all expressed a lot of excitement about this type of caregiving setup. But they also admitted that such programs have not been successful so far. They attributed these failures to a lack of institutional resources to devote to training and programming, which is undoubtedly true. However, I think a key factor that was not mentioned is that so many people in their fifties and sixties—the *dama* generation, in other words—share a skepticism that the state can be depended on to keep its word. As an interlocutor I call Auntie Xiong frankly told me when I asked her if she would consider volunteering for such a program, "You must really think I'm stupid if you think I'm going to spend the last years where I can still move around tending to a bunch of strangers in diapers. I'm going to travel while I still can." Yet another interlocutor, Auntie Song, was even more blunt: "Just do the math," she told me. "There won't be enough people in twenty years. People won't volunteer. Why would they? It'll be even worse when they're the ones needing care." In the absence of the networks of mutual trust and accountability that might exist in a rural village, urban retirees need to believe that the *state* will *ensure* that their volunteer labor is later repaid. The problem is that the state has very little credibility remaining when it comes to asking for sacrifices in exchange for delayed guarantees.

The attitude of "play a day, count a day" is not so much a flippant dismissal of reality but rather a strategy to cope with it. Thomas Malaby (2009) invites us to shift our understanding of play by acknowledging it as a kind of "readiness to improvise in the face of an ever-changing world"(206). This appears to be exactly what the *dama* are doing. In the absence of good solutions—a plan that might work, an assurance that puts worries to rest, a new forecast about the future that can sweeten the bitterness of the past—they simply focus on living well while they still can, however they can. Seen in this light, their seemingly blithe attitudes and devotion to having a good time take on deeper layers of meaning. They like to *shua* because it is all they are guaranteed.

5
The Flavor of Life

I have so far focused my attentions on aspects of post-reform urban life that are shared by, and in many ways particular to, the retired women who participate in congregational dance groups. By highlighting how dance groups figure into retired women's efforts to make sense of the rapidly changing social landscape and carve out spaces where their own needs can be met, I have shown that congregational dancing is not only a symptom of or reaction to these broader social changes. Instead, I have argued that congregational dance groups are venues where retired women can learn, grapple with, and even challenge emerging social norms on their own terms. What still needs to be addressed is the question of why dancing is the medium through which these efforts occur. Why have millions of retired women formed dance groups and not, say, knitting groups, book clubs, or walking meetups? What qualities are inherent to groups organized around dancing that are not present in social organizations of other kinds? If retired women are using these groups as tools with which to navigate post-reform realities, as I have argued, then how are these realities reflected and refracted by dance as an instrument through which social meaning is created and conveyed? I now return to the topic of dancing to confront these questions head-on, and to clarify the stakes of what I have described so far.

During the course of my fieldwork, I was repeatedly struck by how differently congregational dancers and their observers—that is, other urban residents—framed the phenomenon. While urban residents tended to believe that retired women join dance groups to socialize and exercise, which is true, dance group participants tended to place greater emphasis on how much they enjoyed being able to express themselves through the act of dancing. In fact, many people told me that the opportunity to engage in self-expression was what compelled them to join a dance group in the first place. "If it weren't for how I feel when I move to music," a fifty-eight-year-old dance group participant surnamed Zheng told me, "I would just join my husband when he takes his after-dinner walks. That's also exercise. But walking has no flavor." This "flavor," or *weidao*, came up so many times during interviews with congregational dancers concerning their reasons for joining groups that I can confidently assert that for participants, *weidao* is what distinguishes dancing from other available pastimes like playing mahjong or even practicing tai chi.

The concept is difficult to translate into English. Though a dictionary might define *weidao* as taste, flavor, or odor, the word can take on many other meanings in different contexts. When used while appraising a film or musical performance, it might refer to feeling or passion, as in, "The pianist played with much *weidao*." It might also mean beauty when used to describe a place, a painting, or a human being, especially when this beauty has a *je ne sais quoi* quality to it. For example, during a conversation about the British royal family, a friend of mine in Chengdu declared that while he did not find Catherine, the Duchess of Cambridge to be particularly pretty, he did think her *weidao* was exceptional. Finally, it can refer to significance or meaning, such as the time I read a famous Chinese poem in a stone carving at a local park and was forced to admit to my companion that though I understood each individual word, I lacked the literary knowledge to get any *weidao* out of the verses.

All this is to say that when congregational dancers profess to enjoy dancing because it has *weidao*, they are referring to a kind of affective valence that is as powerful as it is ineffable. Along with *duanlian* or *jiansheng* [exercise], *pailian* [rehearse], and *fuzhuang* [costume or outfit], the word is a key part of everyday language of congregational dancing: teachers admonish students to pay attention to the nuances of certain movements lest they get the *weidao* of the dance wrong; members of dance groups disparage other groups for dancing without *weidao*, pieces are chosen for practice or performance for their favorable *weidao*. At a certain point in my research, I began to think of *weidao* as the "substance" of life—that is, an emergent property, particular to each individual object, activity, or situation, that lends interest and meaning to otherwise mundane happenings. Though I met very few dance group participants who were truly proficient dancers in an objective sense, their pursuit and enjoyment of the *weidao* of dance tells me that many congregational dancers savor dancing as a form of creativity. And therein lies the problem.

Creative expression of all kinds—including dance—has occupied an uneasy and at times outright contentious place in Chinese society for hundreds of years, but especially since Mao Zedong took power at the helm of the People's Republic in 1949. It is important to note that in China, the tension between art and politics is not a mere side effect of other policies but rather an intentional feature of the modern nation-state that can be traced to the inception of the Chinese Communist Party itself. Speaking to an audience of literati, artists, and intellectuals at the Yan'an Forum on Literature and Art in 1942, Mao asserted that there is "in fact no such thing as art for art's sake, art that stands above the classes, art that is detached from or independent of politics" (McDougall 1980). The Yan'an Forum played a major role in the consolidation of the Chinese Communist movement under Maoism (as distinguished from Marxism and Leninism), and by using it as a platform, Mao intended to not only clarify the role of artists and literati in the ongoing revolution but also lay the foundation for a new reality in which political ideals superseded artistic freedom. The influence of these words reached its peak when, during the Cultural Revolution, excerpts from the Yan'an speech were quoted in the Little Red Book of Mao's works and used as justification for widespread censorship. Only a few films, books, and so-called revolutionary operas staged by Mao's wife Jiang Qing were deemed to be politically acceptable during this period; all works considered to be "bourgeois"—that is, everything not on that very short list—were banned altogether.

In 1982 the Chinese Communist Party formally revisited the Yan'an Forum and declared Mao's assertion that the only legitimate function of art is in service of socialist political goals to be an "incorrect formulation" (Gladston 2015). However, the idea that art does not and cannot exist for art's sake continues to cast a long shadow over artistic enterprises—from fine art to literature to cinema—in the People's Republic to this day. There are few who would seriously characterize congregational dancing as an art form; I also never met a single *dama* who described herself as an artist or even a *wudaojia*—"[vocational] dancer." And yet, these women's repeated emphasis of the expressive dimensions of the activity cannot be ignored. Their ability to extract something personal and intangible from dancing is in diametrical opposition to government efforts to make the phenomenon into something measurably useful, thus creating a fundamental tension at the heart of congregational dancing.

In what follows, I examine some of the strategies that the state has employed to turn congregational dancing into, to quote Mao at the Yan'an Forum again, a "powerful weapon for uniting and educating the people and for attacking and destroying the enemy... [one that helps] people fight the enemy with *one heart and one mind*" (McDougall 1980, emphasis added). I highlight several cases that demonstrate how various state institutions have attempted to co-opt congregational dancing to promote social harmony and certain kinds of social progress. At the same time, I also contend that dancers have exploited these state agendas for their own benefit. Through the discursive tactics of irony and dismissiveness that many *dama* take on by focusing on leisure, they manage to preserve the *weidao* of congregational dancing without outright resisting or rejecting government interventions. Though dancers and the state actors that seek to regulate them have different agendas, the phenomenon offers both parties a platform from which to assert their interests and broadcast their respective messages to a broad audience. These opposing agendas hang in a delicate balance for the time being.

What is worth thinking about here is not whether the state plays a role in directing how congregational dance groups make their dance selections or perform their pieces. It is indisputable that it does play a role and that this role is expanding. Though the cases I present in this chapter are each windows into the ways in which state actors have inserted themselves into the day-to-day goings-on of dance groups, the fact that the state has an interest in regulating a massive social phenomenon is not in itself remarkable. Rather, I aim to draw attention to how ordinary people learn to express personal meaning in a society where such expression is always subject to scrutiny and control. By doing so, I hope to offer some answers to questions that have hounded me from the very beginning of my research until the present day: How can congregational dancers extract *weidao* from their participation in dance groups when the value of their efforts is ultimately arbitrated by the state? What do they find fulfilling about an activity that is dictated, in so many ways, by people and organizations that have priorities so different from their own? To put it another way, why dance at all?

Case 1: The Twelve Model Routines

On March 23, 2015, the state-run Xinhua News Agency announced a set of new regulations for congregational dancing. Given the scale and disruptiveness of congregational dancing in some public spaces throughout the country, this was hardly surprising. During my preliminary research in Chengdu, I heard repeatedly from both dancers and nondancers alike that some consistent guidelines would be helpful for ameliorating conflict. It might have made a great deal of sense, then, for the central government to set national ordinances on the hours or locations that congregational dancing is permitted, as well as a reliable complaint-reporting mechanism to replace the confusing jumble of police, residential, and commercial security forces that handled conflicts.

In an unanticipated twist, the regulations turned out to address none of these concerns. Instead, the state-run General Administration of Sports (GAS), sponsored by the Ministry of Culture, hired then twenty-nine-year-old national dance competition champion Wang Guangcheng to produce twelve standardized dance routines for all congregational dancing groups to follow (*China Daily*, March 23, 2015). The model routines posted to the web on March 23 show Wang and two backup dancers demonstrating synchronized aerobic dance movements set to contemporary Chinese pop songs. These included the then tremendously popular "Little Apple," an upbeat love song with saccharine-sweet lyrics; a patriotic and catchy number called "Chinese Flavor," by the husband-wife folk-pop duo Phoenix Legend; and the Mongolian-style pop tune "Looking to Beijing from the Grassland." Though Wang does incorporate some stylistic elements into the pieces—for example, a galloping horse motion meant to call pastoral lifestyles to mind in "Looking to Beijing from the Grassland"—for the most part his choreography is simple, streamlined, and easy to learn.

Liu Guoyang, the chief of GAS's mass-fitness department, said in a joint press conference with officials from the Ministry of Culture that public dancing "represents the collective aspect of Chinese culture, but now it seems the over-enthusiasm of participants has dealt it a harmful blow with disputes over noise and venues. So we have to guide it with national standards and regulations" (*China Daily,* March 24, 2015).

> GAS announced on its own website that the standardization of dance routines would take place in three phases over the course of five months, which would ensure "the orderly and scientific development of aerobic dancing" in all 31 provinces (GAS March 25th 2015). The plan was to send 600 dance instructors personally trained by Wang Guangcheng to regional centers and delegated with the task of teaching the routines to leaders of provincial-level dance institutions, who in turn would teach local teachers, and so on and so forth until all dancers were familiar with the official routines. In case there was any confusion about the intent of the model routines, the press release included a statement that read, "From this day forward there will no longer be different dance routines for each community, but instead unified national routines" (*China Daily,* March 24, 2015).

At first glance, these efforts to control the dancers' bodily movements rather than managing the intersection of congregational dancing with other aspects of public life is difficult to understand. The model routines and their proposed implementation resemble something out of a Foucauldian nightmare, with the physical body being disciplined in the service of the body politic. Indeed, the swift and relentless media backlash to the announcement signaled that the state had overplayed its hand. Commentators ranging from anonymous netizens to university professors derided the twelve model routines as having missed the point, with many noting that no one had complained about the quality or content of the dancing (*Christian Science Monitor,* March 24, 2015; op-ed in *People's Daily,* March 27, 2015). A dancer in Beijing told a reporter from the *New York Times* that the regulations would defeat the whole point of congregational dancing, which was that it was "voluntary" and "free," adding that she could not understand why the government needed to get involved at all (*New York Times,* March 24, 2015). Across the Chinese web, commentators began lampooning the government's efforts to manage the dancers, with many insisting that what was really needed to address the dancing "problem" was more alternative recreational activities for retirees to choose from.

In response to this media firestorm, GAS and the Ministry of Culture backtracked from their statements a mere three days after the announcement. In a press release posted on the GAS website and in statements to the *People's Daily* (the official newspaper of the CCP), Liu Guoyang stressed that the twelve model routines were only meant to be suggestions and were in no way intended to replace congregational dancers' own choreography choices. He argued that the concerns voiced by dancers and others on social media were unfounded, and that the whole thing had just been a big misunderstanding (*People's Daily*, March 26, 2015). The Xinhua News Agency also published an announcement clarifying that the model routines were not "mandatory" (March 26, 2015), even going as far as to state, "The era where all people are forced to follow only one orthodox [standard] is long gone and people now require more individualism." To actually enact and enforce standardized dancing on a hundred million congregational dancers, Liu Guoyang insisted, would have been "impossible."

Significantly, the timeline of events suggests that the ministries in question were learning in real time that this was actually impossible. There is simply no way to interpret the March 23 press releases as anything other than an attempt to standardize congregational dancing throughout China. By the time the backlash gained momentum, however, the cat was too far out of the bag for state actors to revise their intentions without losing some face. Nevertheless, the fervor blew over as quickly as it began. When it became apparent that the model routines would have no material impact on anyone's lives, people moved on, and the story all but disappeared from media platforms.

The account I have presented so far is an indisputable case of the triumph of self-determination and creative expression over state overreach. As is often the case, however, media narratives become far more complicated when corroborated with ethnographic data. Three months after these events unfolded, in late June 2015, I arrived in Chengdu in time to ask the members of four different dance groups—a total of approximately sixty people—about their thoughts on the model routines and the fallout that ensued. To my great surprise, only a handful of dancers from each group had even heard of the story. Even more striking was what happened after some discussion among themselves. When everyone was briefed with a synopsis of the March events, the dancers invariably rejected the idea that they were ever in any danger of having their dances standardized by the state. Instead, they suggested that GAS and the Ministry of Culture simply wanted to help them dance in a more attractive manner.

When I asked what they thought of a young state-hired dancer in Beijing determining their dance moves in their own parks and residential complexes, many of my interlocutors expressed some exasperation at the premise of the question. "Of course it's a good thing," a fifty-nine-year-old dance group participant I called Auntie Cai exclaimed. "It means that we have access to higher-quality dancing. It means that the government is taking notice of us!" In her eyes, this form of government interference is not a burden or a method of bodily discipline, but rather a sign that congregational dancing is something worthy of official attention. Once congregational dancing captured the attention of the Beijing Dance Academy, several of my more patient interlocutors explained to me, it became something different altogether: it meant that "they"—presumably the state—did not dismiss the phenomenon because it was dominated by retirees, but rather recognized it as something that is currently relevant and in need of continuing development. It became something officially approved of, thought about, and discussed rather than a bunch of retired women frolicking in the street.

To make sense of why dance participants would so unceremoniously dismiss such credible threats to curtail their creative expression from the central government, it is necessary to first understand that congregational dancing was never a grassroots phenomenon to begin with. A major misunderstanding about congregational dance groups that I often encountered during my research—even among locals who knew someone who participated in a group—was that the dancers choreograph their own routines. This mistake may be explained by significant variations in congregational dancers' technical abilities. It can be difficult to spot similarities or patterns between groups when amateur dancers are just trying to keep up.

The truth is that congregational dance groups seldom, if ever, engage in choreography. Some follow along to videos on portable DVD players, while others are guided by a teacher who learned the dances from another (more experienced) dance teacher or from online videos. While teachers often modify dances in order to match the ability of the participants, a keen observer will notice that dance routines can look remarkably similar across groups. Certain pieces sometimes come into vogue, and on an evening walk around the city one can get a distinct sense of deja vu as one hears the same songs and sees the same routines over and over.

Several dancers I interviewed compared the release of the twelve model routines to a continuing series of official choreography released by the Beijing Dance Academy called the *yangge tao,* or "folk dance sets." Like the twelve model routines, *yangge tao* are choreographed by "expert" dancers expressly for wide distribution and are disseminated to the populace from the center to the peripheries of society. Top teachers from each province are selected to go to Beijing to be taught by the academy choreographer, and the skills trickle down from there. In other words, the proposed mechanisms for spreading the twelve model routines were modeled after processes that were already in place.

In more recent years, this path of dissemination has become even more simplified and streamlined with the rise of online videos and smartphone apps.

When I joined the Dancing Beauties group in 2016 and asked Teacher Yuan whether she ever looked to the *yangge tao* when making decisions about which dances to teach to the group, she enthusiastically replied in the affirmative. She then pulled up a video on her smartphone and asked, "Look familiar?" The video showed four young women performing a Chinese folk dance with traditional silk fans as handheld props; it was the same dance that Teacher Yuan had been teaching to our group for the past few weeks. The title of the video indicated that the dance was from the seventh *yangge tao*. It was unclear whether the four women were from the Beijing Dance Academy or just especially proficient amateurs; in either case, the video had been watched over 600,000 times, and it was evident that the *yangge tao* had a new avenue through which to reach an even wider audience. "I watch these videos all the time!," Teacher Yuan explained. "They're easy to follow, and you can pause them whenever you want if you missed something."

Teacher Yuan is not alone in her proclivity toward online dance videos that originate with the Beijing Dance Academy. Nearly every dance group participant I spoke to on this subject—particularly teachers, group leaders, and women who tend to dance at the front of the pack because they are more confident—reported watching online dance videos on a regular basis. Some of them mentioned the *yangge tao* directly, while others said they did not pay attention to where the videos originated but rather focused on choosing videos that showcased superior dancing—the more *biaozhun* (meaning standard or correct), the better. To put this all another way, dance groups had been looking to "official" dance sources for inspiration and instruction for years prior to the release of the twelve model routines. It made no sense, then, for them to suddenly become up-in-arms over something that so closely resembled what they were already used to.

All this is to say that what many observers—including myself, initially—failed to understand about the March 2015 events was that it was not an instance of state agencies trying to gain control over a social phenomenon for the first time. By hiring a skilled professional to choreograph routines for dances that were popular with congregational dancers, the Ministry of Culture and GAS were merely trying to reform and codify something that was already within its purview. Many congregational dancers find plenty to enjoy about the activity despite—and in some ways because of—the fact that their routines are choreographed by dance experts in Beijing. If anything, they welcome the attention from the central government, since such attention lends their activity a sense of legitimacy and official acceptance. It is in the act of dancing itself, of recalling and performing movement, of aligning one's body with the music, that they get the *weidao* of dance. The creative origins of the routines are beside the point.

This brings me to an additional point about the rollout of the model routines. Prior to my June 2015 visit to Chengdu, I assumed that congregational dancers would be put off by the fact that the Ministry of Culture only provided a dozen routines for them to emulate. Considering that they dance on a nearly daily basis, I was certain that people would exhaust twelve routines in a very short time. This turned out to be a misplaced concern. As I learned more about congregational dancing, I discovered that dance groups generally do not develop extensive repertoires of dance routines. In the year I spent as a full-time member of the Dancing Beauties and Sunset Dance Group, for example, I learned a grand total of two new dances from start to finish—one in each group. Most of the practice time was instead spent on revisiting routines that the group has already learned and mastered. With each practice, people discovered that they had forgotten some bits and needed to brush up, or that they were finally able to get through a difficult part of the dance for the first time. This process was iterative, and though my time as a participant was relatively short, even I began to savor those moments when my feet landed in just the right way after weeks and weeks of missing the mark. Once everyone could dance the whole routine with few mistakes, the group moved on to another number—something that had not been revisited for a few months—and the process started over again.

Perhaps where GAS and the Ministry of Culture went wrong was in attempting to use anachronistic language and procedures to produce their desired results. In the context of the past seventy years of Chinese politics, especially if we recall Mao Zedong's admonition that art needed to help people fight errant ideologies with one heart and one mind, the proposed standardization project was not at all remarkable. During the collective era in general and the Cultural Revolution in particular, group exercise was used to produce healthy, disciplined workers (see Brownell 1995). Revolutionary songs and dancers were popular pastimes, as were soviet-style calisthenics that were often practiced by whole factories and communes before beginning the workday. When congregational dancing began to incite public disorder and complaints on a massive scale, it seems clear that GAS and the Ministry of Culture believed the first step in reasserting control over a massive public phenomenon was to drive it back into this earlier framework of officially sanctioned, officially choreographed collective exercise. However, as I have shown, the ethnographic data suggests that the mechanisms of this control regulation are incredibly mundane, and often occurs with the full consent of the people being regulated because they get something beneficial out of it. The mistake that Liu Guoyang and others made was calling it for what it is: he pulled back the curtain. And even then, many people the policies were aiming at simply shrugged.

Case 2: Dance Competitions and Staging Harmony

In the end, the twelve model routines failed to standardize congregational dancing throughout China. However, this failure was no more than a minor public relations mishap for the Ministry of Culture and GAS. The model routines were neither the first nor sole strategy the state has employed to co-opt the congregational dancing phenomenon; congregational dancers' bodily movements had already been subject to evaluation and regulation from local governing officials well before the March 2015 incident. Though there have always been those who prefer to participate in a version of the phenomenon that precludes state interference (the woman interviewed by the *New York Times* about the twelve model routines comes to mind), the fact remains that efforts to institutionalize congregational dancing have been in place for years, with little fanfare or pushback.

Due to the self-organized nature of the phenomenon and to the scrappy appearance of many groups, the complex links between dancers' desire for recognition and state efforts to impose its will on the phenomenon are easily overlooked. Nowhere are these entanglements more apparent than at local congregational dance competitions (*guangchang wu bisai*), which have been held on a regular basis throughout Chinese cities, including Chengdu, since at least 2009. The competitions are organized in a way that resembles beauty pageants or chess tournaments: the top-ranked groups at the neighborhood (*shequ*) level represent the neighborhood at the sub-district (*jiedao*) level, and the leaders in that competition then advance to the district (*qu*) level, until one group is crowned the winner in a large event that draws contestants from all over the city.

For organizers, such competitions offer opportunities for publicity and network-building. Sponsorship lists for these events often look like a who's who of local power brokers. Competitions are also frequently cosponsored by large corporations and hosted on corporate property. For example, a city district (*qu*)-level competition I attended in 2017 was held on the grounds of a newly opened shopping center owned by the real estate conglomerate Longfor Properties, and the company logo was conspicuously displayed at the event. Other sponsors included the China Sports Lottery, the *jiedao* government, the *qu*'s elderly sports association, and the *jiedao*'s social work organization. Competitions are frequently televised (though aired on peripheral channels and at odd times; I rarely managed to catch them on TV despite my best efforts) and hosted by a sharply dressed MC speaking impeccable standard Mandarin with a knack for riling up the crowd. Finally, these competitions are invariably judged by a panel of government officials, sometimes with input from a professional dancer or choreographer. At the event at the Longfor mall, the most senior official present was the district deputy party secretary, a man in his fifties whose miserably bored expression remained the entire time he was there.

For dancers, these competitions are rare occasions to dance for an audience and to showcase the skills they worked hard to build. If one attends such events in hopes of enjoying a colorful variety of dance styles and performances, however, one would be sorely disappointed. Every group performs a routine that is

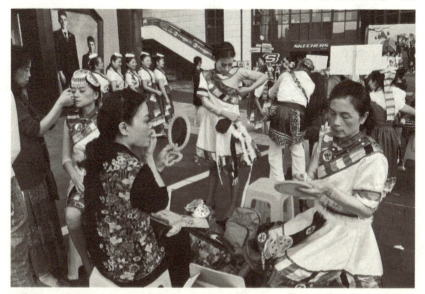

FIGURE 7 Women participating in a dance competition put on Tibetan-style costumes while waiting for their turn to perform. (Photo by Claudia Huang)

preselected by competition organizers and given roughly three months to prepare. At the Longfor mall, where groups from all over the district were vying for a chance to advance to the citywide level competition, the audience was treated to twenty-three incredibly similar renditions of a dance routine set to the Tibetan-style Chinese folk song *"Kangding Qingge"* [*Kangding* Love Song].

When I arrived at the competition on a summer morning, I saw hundreds of middle-aged and older women—along with a few men—sitting together in what looked like a rainbow sea of lustrous polyester. I first approached a group of women all dressed in flamingo-pink robes with yellow-and- green embroidered trim. They were helping each other put on complicated headpieces consisting of plaited ribbons with beading directly over the forehead and long, thin, black braids flowing from the back. They each wore red satin stockings over their shoes to mimic knee-high boots when seen from afar. Directly next to these flamingo-hued dancers sat another group in nearly identical getups, save the fact that theirs were sky-blue instead of pink. Still another group rehearsed nearby. Their costumes consisted of red robes with detachable long sleeves that extended more than twelve inches past their fingertips, as well as a slightly different version of the same headpiece. As each of the groups ascended the stage to perform the same routine in succession, these sleeves and the ubiquitous black braids created graceful shapes in the air as the women danced.

Like the song *"Kangding Qingge"* itself, the costumes that participants wore to the competition are not so much Tibetan as they are Tibetan-esque: though some elements like the long sleeves and the thin braids do appear in traditional Tibetan dress, the outfits are haphazard amalgamations of customary attire from different Tibetan regions and different social classes. When I asked the dancers—all of whom belonged to the majority Han ethnic group—about the origins of what they were wearing, they all answered that they had been purchased online. Indeed, dance costumes like these can be found on China's mega online retailers like Taobao for less than 100 RMB (about 15 USD). Among the striped tracksuits used for aerobics-style dances, the People's Liberation Army uniforms worn in nostalgic performances set to revolutionary-era music, and the red crepe pantsuits with mandarin collars and floral embroidery used in traditional Chinese *yangge* dances, one can also find an entire subcategory of outfits designated for *minzu wu,* or "ethnic dance." From here, the categories become even more specific: Tibetan, Mongolian, Miao, Uighur, and so on. Each of the categories contains costumes that reference key elements of traditional dress from each minority nationality, such as elaborate silver headdresses for Miao outfits and cowboy hats for Mongolian ones.

Again, the vast majority of *dama* spent their youths surviving the brutal excesses of Mao's political campaigns, and then, just as China was transforming into the world's second-largest economy, were squeezed out of their jobs to make way for younger workers. For these women, performing onstage while wearing attention-grabbing costumes can offer a chance to be noticed again after a lifetime of being overlooked. Despite their shoddy construction and cheap materials, the costumes have an ostentatious beauty that is normally deemed immodest for retired women but is sanctioned during performance events such as these dance competitions. Though I personally never participated in a competition, many of my friends and interlocutors did. When I asked my friend Qiu what she enjoyed most about the competitions, she immediately named the outfits—she loved them for their brightness, and for the way they popped in photographs. "At our age," she explained, "the only way to add color to our appearance is with clothing."

Preserving photographic records of these costumes is a requisite feature of dance competitions. After the judging at the Longfor mall had concluded, groups of women gathered onstage to pose for photos in their outfits, taking care to arrange their bodies so as to display the colorful skirts and bright embroidery. For these retirees, dance competitions are performances of visibility. If the cultural insensitivity of the costumes ever gave them pause, they did not voice it. After all, they would be just as happy performing a folk Chinese dance in traditional Han clothing, but that simply is not what the organizers chose.

The fact that organizers chose *"Kangding Qingge"* is neither an accident nor an anomaly. I do not have access to a comprehensive list of competition pieces in Chengdu, but I attended over twenty competitions from 2015 to 2017, and "ethnic minority" dances featured in more than half of them. Tibetan dances were by far the most common, but there were also two Miao dances and a wintertime competition where groups performed a Uighur dance while wearing costumes trimmed with faux fur. For the government agencies that organize them, the dance competitions are public events where ideals—about active aging, about preserving cultural traditions, and in this case, about a unified multiethnic Chinese nation—can be communicated to the masses.

Identifying, categorizing, and codifying ethnic groups was one of the first projects of the new Communist government after the founding of the People's Republic in 1949, and China now officially recognizes fifty-six ethnic groups, including the majority Han. Since 1949, displays of national unity have prominently featured popular understandings of minority groups' cultural heritage. While the state exerts tight control over minority populations' expressions of their own cultural practices, performances of minority songs and dances make regular appearances on state-run television programs, and the idea that China is comprised of fifty-six distinct but harmoniously coexisting ethnic groups remains a foundational tenet of the modern state. Nowhere was this more prominently displayed than during the opening ceremony of the 2008 Olympics, when fifty-six schoolchildren representing the fifty-six ethnic groups carried the Chinese flag into the stadium while wearing versions of traditional attire. In other words, dance competitions that showcase happy elders dancing in Tibetan dress must be understood in the context of this broader tradition of staging national and ethnic harmony. Art, including performance art, in the PRC is always instructive, and one of the enduring lessons of the modern nation-state concerns the inscription and reinscription of the state's borders. On the dance competition stage, the boundaries of the modern Chinese state are asserted through this most visible and, on the balance, most popular officially sanctioned cultural phenomenon to emerge in recent years.

As for *Kangding Qingge* itself, it is commonly performed as a sparse romantic ballad, but the "dance remix" version begins with two slow, dramatic bars prominently featuring a man's voice chanting "Kangding" over the supporting voices of backup singers. An upbeat baseline then abruptly takes over, and the rest of the song is a fast-paced and high-energy number with multiple drum interludes. When the first group at the Longfor mall took the stage, they used the musical introduction to arrange themselves into a clustered formation, smiling steadily while holding the skirts of their Tibetan-style costumes outward to display their colorful patterns. They quickly spread out into two parallel lines facing the audience when the faster portion of the song started. Once in this new formation, they lifted their crossed arms in front of them and swung their hips from side to side to the rhythm of the music. They then added synchronized arm tosses coordinated with leg kicks that consisted of bringing the right foot in front of the body at a forty-five-degree angle. At various points in the routine, the group split into three inward-facing circles while twirling their skirts. Though the full song is about six minutes long with a moment of silence following a climatic denouement in the middle, the dance ended at this midway point to enthusiastic applause. The group descended from the stage, and the host announced the next group, which then ascended the stairs and took position in the same manner as the first group before giving a nearly identical performance.

For over two hours, the twenty-three participating groups performed this shortened version of "*Kangding Qingge*" with minimal variation. Instead of beginning the piece in a clustered formation, some groups chose to start in two parallel lines. In the rare cases where groups had male members, the men appeared onstage donning costumes resembling the traditional garb of Tibetan herders and holding drums. They stood to the sides, drumming rhythmically while the women danced. Two groups performed in matching spandex bodysuits instead of costumes. For the most part, however, any one of the groups' performances could have easily been mistaken for another's. Such repetition failed to sustain the attentions of the audience, which was made up almost entirely of women of all ages (mothers, grandmothers, nannies) with young children, who had all probably wandered by on their morning walks and stopped to check out the commotion. By the tenth performance or so, people had stopped applauding altogether despite increasingly plaintive pleas for enthusiasm from the MC.

What did vary significantly between groups was technical ability. Much like an Olympic event, each performance received a score between 1 and 10 from the judges. At this competition, the lowest score given was 8 and the highest was 9.4. Directly after the performances concluded, the director of a local professional dance academy—a woman in her forties with perfect posture, surnamed Zhou—went onstage to offer feedback to all the participants. She explained that points were deducted for improper movements, for nonmatching costumes, for allowing one dancer to take center stage while the rest of the group performed limited movements, and for not dancing with enough energy. The most significant point deductions, however, were reserved for deviations from the standard [*biaozhun*] routine. She pointed out discrepancies so minor that they had barely registered in my (admittedly untrained) notice during the performances: substituting straight-legged kicks for ones slightly bent at the knee, throwing one arm over the head instead of both arms, twirling the skirts too much, concluding with acrobatic poses, and so on. She gestured to the banner bearing the event's name and reiterated that this was a dance competition, not a choreography competition: the groups, she emphasized, are judged on their ability to faithfully reproduce the official choreography. In her concluding remarks, Ms. Zhou extolled everyone to put more effort into practices and to aim for perfection.

Echoing what happened earlier with the twelve model routines, the dancers I interviewed after Ms. Zhou's remarks were entirely sympathetic to the judging system and thought that they had received the score they deserved. One woman, whose team had received a score of 8.4, told me, "We got such a low score because two of our dancers wore different-colored costumes, and because there were two spots in the song where we had a solo dancer while the rest of us stood in the back barely moving. Zhou said that you can't do this. So we lost points. It's a shame." When I asked the members of another group if they thought it was fair that they were judged according to these criteria, they answered that it would not be a real competition if there were no criteria. They were only disappointed because they had not been informed of the criteria beforehand. "But we know now," a woman surnamed Wei said. "So we won't make the same mistakes again." Like the women who had no qualms with the twelve model routines, Ms. Wei and the others I interviewed all seemed to believe that the competition's officials were simply trying to help them become better dancers. Again, the presence of criteria or standards did not bother them. On the contrary, they understood these standards to be sources of legitimacy and recognition.

Congregational dancing has all the trappings of a grassroots phenomenon. It occurs in public, is mostly self-organized by participants, and has no discernible official agenda. But in many ways, congregational dancing is simply another facet of "official" Chinese dance culture rather than an alternative to it. In her dissertation on dance in the PRC, Emily Wilcox (2011) traces the unusually centralized nature of dance culture and practice in China to the fact that professional dance simply did not exist prior to the formation of the party-state. It was created from scratch under the auspices of the newly formed CCP-led People's Republic. When the Beijing Dance Academy was created in 1954, its curricula and practices became the standard for both provincial dance schools and dance troupes throughout the country (20). Though the retired women who participate in congregational dance groups are not professional dancers and do not aspire to be, they nonetheless think of state-run institutions like the Beijing Dance Academy as the primary if not sole referent for quality and taste.

The relationship between the congregational dancing phenomenon and the state (at all levels) is far more complex than it first appears. While the state attempts to curtail or co-opt the impacts of the phenomenon on daily life, dance group participants also use state attention as leverage for more social visibility as well as recognition and resources. *Dama* who participate in these dance groups are getting far more than just recreation or exercise out of them. They are also places of refuge from difficult family situations, venues for asserting personal preferences, and breeding grounds for ideas about aging to emerge and transform. In other words, urban dance groups offer multiple avenues of meaning-making for their participants, and being held to the standards of the Beijing Dance Academy or the twelve model routines does not detract from those other avenues. The dance groups are deeply embedded in the everyday lives of their participants because they emerged from an everyday context. When the dance competition at the Longfor mall was over, for example, the Dancing Beauties made no changes to their daily practices and exerted no additional efforts to "perfect" their routines. They just went back to doing what they always did. If what the *dama* treasured about participating in dance groups was the *weidao,* or flavor, that it added to their lives, then the aesthetic dimensions was one of many ingredients. Dance groups existed in urban areas before the state made concerted efforts to co-opt the phenomenon, and by then the *dama* had a major head start in defining the terms of participation.

What would happen, then, when the state has the chance to impose its own terms from participants from the beginning? I had the unexpected opportunity to see for myself when my family took a trip to my grandmother's natal village of Nanchun.

Case 3: Nanchun Village
Nanchun village is a mid-sized agricultural community with about 200 households located on the southern edge of the fertile Chengdu plain. It produces fruits, vegetables, and Sichuan peppercorn on a rolling basis throughout the year, meaning there is hardly any downtime between harvests. Though there are plenty of women of *dama* age, there was no culture of group dancing in Nanchun outside of special holidays. This makes sense when considering the economic underpinnings of congregational dancing. The urban phenomenon is a by-product of economic policies that put millions of people out of work while they were still able-bodied, but the women in Nanchun can hardly be considered "retired" because they typically work until injury or illness prevents them from continuing. Because congregational dancing provides an alternative to idleness—a problem people in agricultural communities seldom have—it never really caught on in the village the way it did in major cities.

But in the spring of 2012, local party cadres decided that it was high time for Nanchun women to start dancing like their urban counterparts. They approached two women who were well known and respected in the village, handed them 2,000 RMB, and instructed them to use the money to begin a dance group. The money was to be spent on a portable DVD player, speakers, instructional dance videos, and costumes for inter-village dance competitions—which are organized and put on by CCP leaders in each respective village. The cadres even went so far as to secure the local primary school courtyard as the dance venue. Other villagers were quickly recruited, and nightly dancing commenced soon after. By the time I first visited the village in the summer of 2014, the dance group had become a salient social force. When I visited again in 2016 and 2017, even more dancers had joined the group, and heading down to the schoolyard to watch the dancers had become a popular after-dinner activity for many villagers.

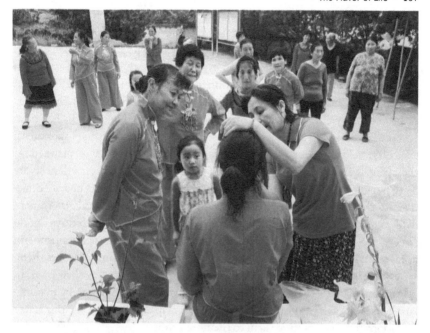

FIGURE 8 Village women help each other apply makeup before dance practice while children look on in Nanchun. (Photo by Claudia Huang)

I have so far been unable to determine the original source of the order to start a dance group in Nanchun, but judging by the level of organization that goes into the inter-village competitions, designs to insert organized dancing into rural life arose from at least the county, if not from the provincial level of government. When I asked one of the village women why she thought the cadres had initiated dancing when they did, she repeated what the cadres had told her when she asked them the same question: "We have a good society now; we can afford to have a little fun."

Though they favor some of the same music and dancing that is popular in Chengdu and throughout China (I was treated to a particularly spirited performance of "Little Apple" during my 2017 visit; by then I had learned the moves with the Sunset Dance Group so I danced along), the impetus behind the formation of these dance groups is diametrically opposite to those in the city. Community-level (*shequ*) officials have begun organizing dance groups in cities in more recent years, but the vast majority of urban groups remain self-organized. Even if there is a paid teacher, she (and it is almost always she) is usually a fellow retiree who dances as a hobby and is treated as a friend or perhaps a mentor, but not necessarily a social superior. In Nanchun village, however, two older male cadres—whom the dancers call "teachers" out of deference—supervise the dance sessions on a frequent basis but never participate in the dancing itself. The dancers select the routines they want to learn from their DVD collection most of the time, but when it comes time to prepare for the inter-village competitions, it is the male "teachers" who choose which dances are performed.

In other words, while the dance group in Nanchun looks a lot like any group one might see in a park in Chengdu, down to their outfits and their choreography, everything else about the congregational dance phenomenon has been co-opted and reimagined by government actors. However, everyone I spoke to in the village told me that they were happy to have an evening activity planned for their benefit and at no cost to themselves. This is not at all to say that dancers are mere puppets of the state, or even that they are passive recipients of state directives. In the case of the village dance group, it is true that the local government deployed congregational dancing as a surrogate for the post-reform "good society"—a shorthand for development, modernity, and cosmopolitanism—in a feat of small-scale social engineering. But it is also true that the dancers themselves have wholeheartedly embraced congregational dancing as their own. In other words, just as the state attempts to control the phenomenon by manipulating its semiotic valences, so do dance participants manipulate the state's intentions by reinterpreting them to their own ends.

Instructing Art, Creating *Weidao*

In an early study on art education in post-reform China published in the late 1980s, psychologist Ellen Winner makes several observations about how Chinese children are taught various types of visual art ranging from Chinese ink drawing to Western-style painting to calligraphy. First, she notes that classes are teacher-oriented, with students learning by emulating the teacher rather than by working together or through trial and error. Teachers demonstrate certain techniques, and students strive to copy that technique as perfectly as possible. Instead of discovering for themselves how certain brush strokes create shapes, students "learn what the masters have already discovered" (1989, 48). Second, Winner writes that Chinese art education is heavily uniform, with art teachers across the country using the same textbooks, which in turn contain the same schemas and models for students to copy. Third, children are not taught to solve "visual problems" on their own. While students are praised for linking discrete skills together—for example, drawing a chicken standing under some grapes after separate lessons on drawing chickens and grapes—any further deviation from the taught standard is understood to be incorrect rather than creative.

"The goal," Winner writes, "is to master the tradition, not to start a new one" (61). In her analysis, Winner posits that Chinese art education focuses almost exclusively on the aesthetic and moral dimensions of art. Under this framework, art is something that is both beautiful and pleasant as well as a medium through which moral values can be communicated. It is not, however, understood as a form of emotional expression or as a vehicle for cognitive development.

At first glance, these observations seem to be deeply rooted in Western stereotypes about Chinese approaches to both education and art: Chinese students are taught to memorize but not to think critically; Chinese people excel at replication but not innovation. However, Winner's argument has less to do with Chinese students' inherent abilities and more to do with how teachers—guided and constrained by state agendas—emphasize and cultivate certain skills over others. Winner situates these observations within the larger context of Chinese society at the time, and notes that what happens within the walls of art classrooms seems to mirror the general social milieu. Chinese society has changed dramatically in the years since Winner conducted her study, and indeed, art education has changed as well.

In *Creativity Class,* Lily Chumley (2016) notes that contemporary Chinese art students are very much preoccupied with cultivating personal styles, and that teaching students to "solve visual problems," so to speak, is now a top priority in art education curriculums. While it would be tempting to attribute these changes to a gradual withdrawal of state influence from art instruction as a result of opening up and reform, Chumley asserts that the exact opposite has occurred. In its efforts to transition the Chinese economy away from manufacturing and toward an information economy in the 2000s, the state began to value innovation and entrepreneurship in workers. Rather than making sure that students come away with a mastery of traditional techniques, arts educators and art schools began to cultivate a new class of "culture workers" who could become the movers and shakers of China's new entrepreneurial economy. What remains the same, however, is the fact that these priorities were set by the state. In other words, it is not that standardization was pushed aside to make way for creativity, but rather that creativity itself has become the standard.

The co-option of artistic practices for a political agenda is not limited to the visual arts (cf. Anagnost 1997; Law and Ho 2011). It is also nothing new, and certainly not a novel invention by the Chinese Communist Party; in fact, we risk losing sight of the broader context of how politics and art intersect in Chinese society if we only look to CCP attitudes and policies as a baseline for comparison. In *Opera and the City* (2012), historian Andrea Goldman argues that in late imperial China, members of the Qing court and other elites transformed Beijing opera from the bawdy, chaotic affairs they once were into orderly and moralistic stagings of Confucian values. These efforts to co-opt the genre—to turn opera performances into mediums for disseminating moral values—were so successful that enforcement was no longer necessary by the end of the Qing dynasty (242). The tastes of the Qing court had become the tastes of the people. Without knowing the history of how these tastes were cultivated and the enforcement that occurred to bring them about, latter-day observers of Beijing opera may well mistake the Confucian moralism often seen in opera performances for "*description* rather than *prescription*" (246; emphasis in original).

There are two main parallels between the historical co-option of Beijing opera and contemporary state efforts to regulate congregational dancing. The first is that in both cases, the state relied on sponsorship and patronage of favored performance pieces rather than outright censorship of unacceptable ones. The second is that despite these efforts to co-opt the genre, there remains room for complexity and nuance in individual performances. This all leads me to the main point concerning the relationship between how art forms are instructed or prescribed and how they are practiced or interpreted: in the same way that congregational dance groups are not entirely "grassroots" or "voluntary," the Chinese state—with the Cultural Revolution period being a probable exception—is also not entirely hegemonic in how it exerts its will. For example, Goldman explains that even as the Qing court attempted to rid Beijing opera of lewd or sexual themes, certain plays with sexual content were nevertheless permitted so long as the sexuality was condemned or moralized. Whether audiences paid closer attention to the sexual content or to the moral narrative is another question altogether.

Similarly, the Ministry of Culture–sponsored twelve model routines may have been intended to foster the "orderly and scientific" development of congregational dancing, but dance group participants paid little attention to the standardization effort and simply appreciated the routines for their attractive choreography. At congregational dance competitions, state organizers may have selected minority nationality dance forms to reassert the boundaries of the nation-state to include contested territories, but the participants were only interested in the attractive costumes and dance moves. In Nanchun, local cadres started dance groups for the sake of adhering to a post-reform development narrative, but the village women mostly enjoyed the dancing as a social pastime. In other words, standardizing the way that an art form is disseminated does not translate to standardized experiences.

I can further clarify this point by sharing my own experiences with art education in China. Like many parents who wanted to give their only child every advantage possible in the increasingly competitive post-reform society, my parents enrolled me in piano lessons before I began primary school. I remember having an unpleasant time at these lessons: my stern, though not unkind teacher taught me two classical pieces at a time (always Bach, Beethoven, Chopin, or Mozart), and I practiced these pieces for hours each day. My teacher assessed my mastery of these pieces at our weekly lessons and either taught me two more if she thought I was ready to move on or sent me home to practice for another week. I was not taught scales, chords, or any kind of musical theory. I was never asked what type of music I preferred or whether I enjoyed certain pieces over others. At least at that level, the goal was never to train me to develop musical taste or to compose anything on my own. Once a year, my parents took me to a citywide piano-credential testing event to determine my playing "level." Like the congregational dance competitions, piano examination participants were given pieces to prepare well in advance and played in front of a panel of judges who determined whether the examinee has passed based on a points system. I was much, much older when I learned that different pianists could have different "interpretations" of the same piece.

As I aged into adulthood, however, I discovered that this highly standardized and uninspiring learning experience taught me more than I had previously believed. As an adult, I developed an appreciation for classical piano music that was undoubtedly informed by my earlier exposure. I found that I could fill in the gaps in my musical education with some personal effort, and that the technical skills I learned as a child served as a foundation for other kinds of knowledge. In other words, the standardized education I received did not ultimately prevent me from developing a different and more nuanced relationship with piano.

Learning to dance with congregational dancers offered a parallel experience. In the Sunset Dance Group weekly class led by Teacher Yuan, I initially felt awkward about the way she incessantly corrected my posture, movements, and comportment. I especially disliked the stretches and exercises that opened each class because it seemed like their goal was to mold my body into specific shapes without consideration for my (or anyone else's) natural strengths or weaknesses. We practiced the same dance routines week after week, often focusing on a single phrase of choreography for hours at a time. I did not grasp the significance of Teacher Yuan's avid consumption of professional dance videos from the *yangge tao* and other officially sanctioned choreographers until I was her dance pupil. She settled for nothing less than the standard version of the routines we practiced: every movement was scrutinized for its accuracy, and each error was dissected and broken down until it was well understood by each of us. At the end of each class, Teacher Yuan exhorted us to watch videos of professional dancers performing the same routine so that we might internalize their movements.

My first few months with the dance group were admittedly difficult: the class felt uninteresting and uninspiring. I repeatedly wondered why we couldn not make room for more self-expression, especially because all of us were only there for personal enjoyment. But with each passing week, my friendships with the other women in the group became deeper, I became more comfortable and familiar with the structure of the class, and though I never truly mastered any of the dances, I performed them with more ease. As the class made more sense to me, it also became more enjoyable. It began to dawn on me that the others in the group loved Teacher Yuan's class precisely because she held them to high expectations and expected them to aim for professional-quality dancing.

By the end of my time in Chengdu, I had begun to look forward to the dance class each week and even found myself defending it to some of my same-generation peers. When a new acquaintance asked me what I thought about the "old fashioned, boring dances" that congregational dancers favored, I replied, to my own surprise, that "I actually think the dances have a lot of *weidao*!" The acquaintance seemed puzzled, and pressed me to clarify, but I could not come up with a satisfactory answer at the time. In retrospect, I believe what I meant was that the dance classes offered me so much by way of exercise and friendship that these enjoyable elements had become melded together with the dance routines themselves. In my mind, they were no longer discrete elements but rather parts of the same flavorful whole.

Regulating Flavor

Most ordinary people I spoke to in Chengdu about the congregational dancing phenomenon agreed that retirees needed something to do to fill their ample time. For them, the fact that so many retired women have chosen to dance is merely incidental, or else simply because people of their generation enjoy collective activities. What many observers who do not participate in congregational dancing overlook is the fact that even recreational activities are not meaningful unless something is at stake. Women who participate in congregational dancing emphasize repeatedly that they are not simply looking to waste time; they are also working to cultivate meaning, interest, and *weidao* in the remaining years of their lives, and dancing is one of the ways they are accomplishing this goal.

I have laid out the ways in which state actors have attempted to co-opt the congregational dancing phenomenon from the top down, as well as the ways in which the phenomenon's participants have reinterpreted and reframed the state's efforts to suit their own interests. I have also argued that a dance group need not be wholly "voluntary" for it to become a venue for self-cultivation and for exploring individual identities: because the state remains the arbiter of legitimacy for ordinary people living in China today, it makes sense that participants pay attention to the standards set by state officials concerning what the dances ought to look like. Striving for and meeting official standards is not solely what they get out of their participation, of course, but standardization and regulation are so much part of the normal fabric of everyday life in China that they are not necessarily roadblocks to other ways of relating to the activity. For now, the two diametrically opposed forces acting on the phenomenon have struck a delicate balance.

One question remains unanswered: "So what?" Even if the dancers can enjoy congregational dancing on their own terms as long as they do so within the confines of state-sanctioned frameworks, the facts remain that congregational dancers in the People's Republic of China are not unified, have no leadership, and have certainly made no political demands. It is an identifiable social phenomenon by outside observers and by the participants' own estimation, but it is also not a cohesive collective in any practical sense. What, then, are the implications of its existence for Chinese society as a whole?

One way to begin to make sense of this question is through the lens of the revival of civil society in the People's Republic. Robert Weller (1999) has written extensively on this subject in his comparisons between Taiwanese and Chinese societies. In this chapter, I have been primarily concerned with highlighting the tensions between the state's efforts to remake the phenomenon into a useful social tool for promoting various agendas and participants' efforts to use dance groups as vehicles of individual expression, as well as highlighting how these two forces interact in the everyday goings-on of the phenomenon. I am aware, however, that another issue lurks beneath the surface: in Weller's prescient words, the real question is not whether large-scale social movements outside of the official state apparatus are possible in post-reform China (I contend that the existence of the congregational dancing phenomenon clearly indicates that they are), but rather, "when those alternatives can coalesce into something able to exert political pressure" (58). It is beyond the scope of this book to answer this question in full, though I do present some possibilities in the next and final chapter. In any case, I offer it as a provocation for thinking about the possible implications of congregational dancing.

The CCP has not tolerated large-scale civil organizations after 1989 (Weller 1999, 57), but has seemed to tolerate congregational dancing so far because it does not present a threat. It is difficult to say how long this tolerance will last. State actors are obviously eager to harness congregational dancing as a tool for their own agendas. There are also signs that as the phenomenon matures, it will become an increasingly regulated and ritualized part of the social landscape. When I was in Chengdu interviewing congregational dance group members about the twelve model routines in the summer of 2015, for example, I also spoke with a mid-level municipal bureaucrat who told me that new housing developments in the city often include specially demarcated space for congregational dance groups, and that in his opinion, "dancing is better than protesting." This ostensibly captures the official government stance on congregational dancing. It suggests that the central government is willing to tolerate dancing—even on the scale of a hundred million participants throughout the country—as long as it does not threaten social harmony. There is also evidence that state actors are prepared to take drastic measures to regulate the phenomenon at the first sign of serious unrest. Though the proposed twelve model routines never became standard following severe media backlash in 2015, the nature of these regulations reveals that it is the individualized character of congregational dancing that has been identified as a threat: what it seeks to control is not the groups' size or public behavior, but rather the bodily comportment and expression of each individual dancer. In other words, the *weidao* of dance—the very thing that dancers cite as the distinguishing characteristic of the activity—is also what threatens the phenomenon's continued proliferation in the future. The fact that the Ministry of Culture attempted to standardize dance routines for all groups across the nation indicates that the relative autonomy enjoyed by congregational dancers cannot be taken for granted.

Finally, as the Nanchun village case shows, state actors will not hesitate to reclaim preexisting forms of sociality to serve their own agendas. It remains to be seen whether city and provincial officials will attempt similar tactics to manipulate the semiotic valences of the phenomenon in urban settings. If and when such a time does come, the present balance between dancers' subjective enjoyment and pursuit of dance's *weidao* and official attempts to regulate the phenomenon from the top down will be disturbed. How such a disturbance will affect congregational dancing—and the relationship between its participants and the state—remains an open question.

Conclusion
● ●

In retrospect, the years when I conducted most of my fieldwork constituted something of a second golden age of China's post-reform era. If the decade of the 1980s was marked by political thaw (especially when measured against the preceding two decades), then the early to mid-2010s were characterized by soaring standards of living and a sort of frenzied optimism. A new skyscraper or bullet train route seemed to be completed on a weekly basis. More and more international companies entered the Chinese market, making previously inaccessible products readily available (and increasingly affordable) to Chinese consumers. For those with steady jobs or steady pensions, life in the major cities felt convenient, efficient, and comfortable. Moreover, there was a palpable sense of possibility and optimism permeating the air. During my time in Chengdu, friends and acquaintances often asked me whether my parents or I regretted leaving China in the 1990s. Some would not accept my equivocations for an answer: they were proud of China's recent achievements and resolutely believed China would dominate the next century. The trade-off that urbanites were asked to make—sacrificing certain individual liberties in exchange for economic growth—seemed like a worthy one to many people. In this sense, my interlocutors' proclamations about good fortune, or being the luckiest generation of Chinese women to have ever lived, fell very much in line with the prevailing attitude of the times.

Things are quite different now. In the last few months of my time in the field, during the lead-up to the Nineteenth National Communist Party Congress in October 2017, hints about impending changes in state-society relations began to emerge in everyday life. The first clue was increased censorship and regulation of speech on social media. WeChat has never been a space for unregulated speech: news items and commentary that criticize the CCP or put the government's actions in a bad light are monitored and taken down even if these conversations take place within contained group chats (Harwit 2016). But in 2017, a new policy was instituted that made group administrators (usually people who began the group or those who had control to approve new members) responsible for content posted in the group. Auntie Wang, the administrator of the Sunset Dance Group's WeChat account, messaged everyone to ask members to refrain from posting any messages of a political or sensitive nature. The group's chats only rarely contained posts on such matters, usually in the form of tongue-in-cheek memes or jokes, but after this warning they disappeared altogether.

The general atmosphere became more tense during this period. Interlocutors and friends often sent me WeChat links to articles and news items related to the congregational dancing phenomenon, retirement, and eldercare. In the fall of 2017, the contents of these links began to disappear with alarming regularity despite the fact that they usually contained nothing more than news reports or light social commentary. I would either receive an error message once I clicked on them, or I would simply never receive the message at all. Sometimes, I would only hear about them when the sender asked me why I never responded. The Chengdu Old Age University, which I had visited dozens of times and where the security guards recognized me by sight, requested that I procure an updated letter of introduction from Sichuan University (my host university) detailing my exact course of study. Dance groups that had ties to local government offices also began to experience intense political outreach efforts. For example, the Sunset Dance Group was summoned to the *shequ* office to watch the opening ceremony of the Party Congress on the office's big screen. It was framed as an invitation to a voluntary community event, but once they arrived, the women were told to pay full attention to the speeches and refrain from using their phones or chatting among themselves. Several people in the group remarked afterward that it felt like the Cultural Revolution again.

Some of this increased censorship and scrutiny was likely episodic in nature and linked directly to the Nineteenth Party Congress (see Ruan et al. 2020), but any subsequent reprieve was short-lived. The COVID-19 pandemic that began in Wuhan in late 2019 introduced such dramatic changes to urban life in China that it will take many years to take full stock of the consequences. The pandemic disrupted people's daily routines throughout the world, but China's "Zero Covid" virus containment strategy took government intrusion into private life to an unprecedented level.

Beginning in the early months of 2020, local governments throughout China began to require citizens to display quick-response (QR) health codes to gain entry into public spaces. Each person had to download the app from WeChat or Alipay (another popular payment, shopping, and lifestyle platform) on a smartphone. The app records people's self-reported symptoms and travel history and tracks people's movement in real time. The app then produces a QR code that turns green, yellow, or red depending on one's degree of COVID-19 exposure. While the rules could vary by location and changed somewhat during the pandemic, green codes were generally required for entry into most public spaces. People received a yellow or red code when they came into contact with (or in some cases merely crossed paths with) a person with the virus, and they were required to stay home or report to a quarantine center. Because the tracking system was live, codes could change at any time, like when one was trying to board a bus or about to enter a store. While no one wanted to be sent to a quarantine center by themselves, anxiety and fear were particularly palpable among older adults who depended on family members for care (see Khan 2022; Stevenson 2022).

The technological disruptions to older adults' senses of autonomy and community also need to be emphasized. As I have previously noted, many urban retirees and all of my interlocutors own smartphones and use them on a daily basis. Many functions of modern living (like paying utility bills or buying train tickets) were long ago integrated into WeChat and Alipay. Despite this previous familiarity with cellular technology, relying on the health code app for mobility and access proved to be difficult for many older adults I know. Several people told me they had trouble with the complicated app interface and sometimes gave up on a planned excursion because they could not get it to work. Researchers have found that older adults oftentimes lost the ability to use public transportation, and therefore much of their mobility, either because they did not have smartphones or because they could not use the health code app (Liu et al. 2021). In my own family's WeChat group, older relatives constantly asked the younger ones for help. They were actually better off than most: according to nationwide surveys, only about 18 percent of adults over age sixty-five use smartphones on a regular basis (Chi, n.d.).

Because so many older adults in China participate in congregational dancing and other group-based activities as their main source of exercise and social connection, social distancing mandates proved to be detrimental to their physical and mental health. Many reported experiencing depressive symptoms and a sense of alienation during the quarantine period in the early weeks of the pandemic, and the prevalence of mental health disorders such as anxiety, depression, and suicide ideation among older adults increased compared with the pre-pandemic baseline (Chen, Chen, and Zhong 2022; Liu et al. 2022). Researchers have also noted that physical activity among older adults noticeably declined during the pandemic, with 67.2 percent of people over age sixty-five describing themselves as "physically inactive" in 2020, compared to just 46 percent in 2018 (Zhou et al. 2022). Congregational dance groups and other common-interest groups are a key source of personal connection and meaning for China's retirees, and being deprived of them even for short periods can bring about feelings of helplessness.

I certainly saw these national trends play out among my interlocutors and friends in Chengdu. During the early months of the pandemic, many older adults I know posted about their frustration, worry, and desperation on WeChat. Qingyi and Liwei, who both focused their social lives around their dance groups, also began to post videos of themselves dancing in their living rooms to pass the time. During the course of the past few years, I heard about various pandemic-related frustrations from my interlocutors, from being called upon to help with childcare for weeks at a time during school closures, to being trapped at home during lockdowns without access to fresh food or fresh air, to feeling panicked about catching the virus during the early weeks of 2023 when the central government abruptly abandoned virus containment measures, resulting in massive spikes in COVID cases throughout China.

COVID-19 upended the two groups that were the focus of my research. When pandemic lockdowns began in the early months of 2020, the dance studio that housed the Dancing Beauties' weekly practices temporarily shuttered its doors. The owner took this opportunity to renovate the building, extending the duration of the hiatus. The building reopened in late 2020 under a significantly different business model: studio rooms were no longer rented by the hour, and individual monthly memberships were required from everyone wishing to use the space. The new pricing structure was cost-prohibitive for the Dancing Beauties. A few people expressed interest in looking for a new venue, but nothing ever came of it. What was meant to be a months-long hiatus turned into an indefinite one. Sadly, the social aspects of the group seem to have fallen by the wayside as well. Between 2020 and 2023, the once-active Dancing Beauties WeChat became noticeably quieter over time. The last time communication in the WeChat group occurred was in January 2023, when a few people posted well-wishes for the Chinese New Year Holiday. No one has said anything ever since.

The Sunset Dance Group fared a little better. The group temporarily disbanded during the initial COVID lockdown but began holding regular practices again in summer 2020. However, the group has become something quite different in the past few years. For one, it is smaller. Several people in the group never returned when the practices resumed. They also stopped participating in the WeChat group. I am not personally close with any of the women who left so did not have a chance to ask about their reasoning, but my educated guess is that tightening social circles and increasing interdependence with kin networks figured into their decisions. The organizing structure of the group has also changed. In May 2021, I awoke one morning to see that I had been removed from the Sunset Dance Group WeChat group. I sent a message to Wenxie, with whom I maintained regular contact, to inquire about what had happened. After several days, she replied that everyone who was not currently attending daily dance practices had been removed. There were now only seventeen people in the WeChat group; previously there were more than thirty. Wenxie was apologetic and seemed a little sheepish, explaining that Auntie Wang wanted to do things more officially. When I asked whether the *shequ* officials were still part of the group chat, Wenxie replied that one of the officials was now a co-administrator of the group. "It's more convenient this way," she wrote, "since we do so many activities with the *shequ* now."

When I texted with Teacher Yuan directly at the end of 2022, she told me that the Dancing Beauties never officially disbanded. People still get together in smaller groups for meals and outings, and there are no hard feelings between anyone. When I asked if she thought that the group might find another studio space or even meet in a public park somewhere, she gave me a noncommittal answer. "The classes were a good thing," she wrote in her message. "But I'm so busy with other things. I'm still dancing, and many of the others are too. We still meet, we still dance, just not together. It's fine like this for now." Teacher Yuan still take classes at the old age university, still travels as much as possible, and still refuses to take care of her granddaughter for more than a few hours a week.

To be clear, the pandemic did not put an end to the congregational dancing phenomenon—far from it. Public spaces throughout China are still filled with the sight and sound of dance groups. According to friends in Chengdu, some groups in certain neighborhoods disappeared, but new ones popped up either in their place or nearby. In a sign of dancers' continued exuberance, the central government passed the first nationwide noise ordinance law targeted at congregational dancers in late 2021 ("Our Country Is Enacting Legislation," 2021). What is undeniable, however, is that the phenomenon is different from what it was when I started this research, and the uneasy status quo that existed for Chinese retirees during the boom years is now once again being renegotiated.

The Zero Covid policy did significant damage to China's economy, with the housing market in crisis and the unemployment rate for young people hitting unprecedented highs. Some observers claim that the fallout marks the "end of China's economic miracle" (Posen 2023). If some *dama* were already anxious and resentful about their prospects when the economy was booming, then their discontent has surely grown since this turning of the tide. For many, the promise of a better future for their children outweighed any complaints they had about the hardships they suffered in their youths or the anxiety they have about their old age. Now that the promise is uncertain, however, the calculus is suddenly very different. I have heard a few grumblings here and there, but none of my interlocutors has openly voiced discontent with Xi Jinping or his policies. I know now to not take their silence at face value.

The past few years have been intense and trying in so many ways for older people living in China. I am not surprised that some groups, like the Dancing Beauties, did not make it through the pandemic. Nor am I surprised that some groups, like the Sunset Dance Group, morphed into something quite different. Because the fact is, the congregational dancing phenomenon was never a stable social object. It was, and is, a symptom of a kind of new attitude about getting older that was set in motion by historical events and will continue to manifest and evolve in various contexts.

Congregational dancing has thrived under a very particular set of social, economic, and political circumstances. The SOE reforms that laid off millions of people from public-sector jobs starting in the late 1990s, combined with compulsory retirement ages that force women out of the workforce at age fifty or fifty-five, produced an enormous pool of urbanites who have little to do with their time despite being physically healthy and active. Many people who were laid off due to SOE reforms formed dance groups, and people who retired in the following years joined these groups upon leaving the work force. Had these reforms not occurred, or had the age of retirement been set even slightly higher, congregational dancing likely may have never reached the critical mass to become a national phenomenon. Moreover, the retirees who participate in congregational dancing are not merely out of work; they are at *leisure*. China's public pension program guarantees former work unit employees a set income (based on salary prior to retirement) for life.

While it is true that most urban retirees cannot afford to live luxurious or privileged lives on these pensions, the guaranteed monthly income allows them to spend at least part of their time on hobbies like dancing rather than devoting all their waking hours to working to make ends meet. Last and perhaps most significantly, the congregational dancing phenomenon can only exist in its current form because the state allows participants the freedom to gather in public in large groups. None of these factors can be taken for granted. The COVID-19 pandemic has certainly increased government scrutiny of group gatherings, but the other conditions that allowed congregational dancing to thrive are also under threat.

In recent years, there have been persistent reports that the central government in Beijing plans to raise the retirement age sometime in the near future to ameliorate the effects of the aging population on China's development trajectory (Beland and Ka 2004; Zhu and Walker 2018). Though such policies have been piloted in a few provinces with mixed success (Hu et al. 2023), it is all but inevitable that people will soon be expected to work longer, decreasing the number of active, independent years they have to spend on recreational activities. The future of the pension program for retired urban workers is also in question. Many smaller reforms to the program have occurred over the past two decades, and so far their effects have been unevenly distributed across income brackets (Smyth 2000; Zhu and Walker 2018). Multiple provinces have forecast that their pension programs will run at deficits as early as 2022, and the northeastern Heilongjiang Province has already been forced to delay pension payments to retirees after being unable to come up with sufficient funds (Rothschild 2019). Practically speaking, I heard from many retirees that their pensions were not keeping pace with the rising costs of living and that they had doubts about whether their pensions could support them as they aged out of independence. More than one interlocutor told me in explicit terms that they plan to dance only until they or their spouses get ill.

All this is to say that the conditions that make congregational dancing possible are fragile. It is likely that changes in any one of the factors will significantly alter the shape and scope of the phenomenon. For now, however, dance groups continue to offer retirees a space to exercise and socialize, and congregational dancers continue to use their groups as venues for cultivating individual interests, extra-familial support networks, and senses of personal enjoyment or *weidao*. That said, I believe that broader implications of congregational dancing transcend the parameters of the phenomenon itself. Even if my own rather pessimistic prognosis about the eventual demise of congregational dancing comes to pass, the phenomenon will already have made an indelible mark on Chinese society. What will remain unchanged is that women of the "lost generation" have discovered the space and opportunity to pursue meaningful aging on their own terms. Already, congregational dancers have taught the Chinese public that elders may have their own consumer tastes and interests distinct from those of the youth, that retirees do not always prefer to retreat into quiet family lives, and most importantly, that there is more than one way to grow old. These are remarkable accomplishments for a segment of society that many people were willing to write off as vestiges of the collective era who cannot think for themselves.

The congregational dancing phenomenon is not simply about how retired people dance. It is also about how they live. Congregational dancing has become an increasingly significant cultural touchstone in China since I began this project nearly ten years ago. By the end of my fieldwork, nearly everyone I met knew somebody who was dancing in a group, and even those who did not had something to say about the phenomenon. Congregational dancers, and the subculture they have created among and for themselves, now appear to be a permanent fixture in the Chinese urban social landscape. On television and the internet, the *dama* are prominently featured in social commentary and comedy sketches poking fun at retirees' habits and behaviors. Shops, online retailers, and beauty salons have begun to cater to the dancers' tastes, hawking colorful wares labeled as *dama* shoes, *dama* clothes, and even *dama* haircuts. Yet despite its visibility and notoriety, I have intentionally avoided treating the phenomenon as a spectacle, choosing instead to highlight the ways in which congregational dancing has been woven into the fabric of everyday life in post-reform China.

Throughout this book, I chose to focus on stories that showcase how the congregational dancing phenomenon figures into retired women's daily lives rather than its sensational and at times disruptive dimensions. I did not, for example, dwell on the conflicts between dance groups and other urban residents over noise or use of public space. Nor did I go into much detail about the props, music, and dance movements of the groups. This is not because I find the conflicts between dancers and other urban residents to be unremarkable, nor is it because I am uninterested in props and music. A group of retirees dancing in sync while wearing matching outfits and holding fans or scarves or even tennis rackets is an undeniably memorable sight. However, what made the deepest impression on me as I conducted research on congregational dancing is not the dancers' colorful accessories or the sight of hundreds of retired women filling a city square, but rather the fact that ordinary people are trying to make sense of rather extraordinary circumstances through the act of coming together and dancing.

I began this project because I, like so many others who have observed them with a passing glance, was charmed and bemused by the so-called dancing grannies. I expected to find that the dance groups function as a source of camaraderie for people who lack access to official sources of sociality such as jobs or civil associations. These predictions turned out to be true in many ways, but they did not capture a complete picture. As the dancers invited me into their groups and into their world, I also bore witness to their frustrations with state policies that by turns patronized and neglected them, as well as their bewilderment with their children's changing priorities. I did not expect to find that dance groups would play a central role in helping people navigate these shifting post-reform realities: dance groups are simultaneously venues where retirees can practice self-cultivation, spaces for living out a new form of old age that emphasizes individual responsibility, incubators where new ideas about what it means to be a grandparent can emerge, and a testing ground for the state's ambitions to provide all citizens with the "good life" while maintaining social harmony.

I also did not expect to find dance group participants to be, for the most part, so utterly enchanted with this new phase of their lives. In the empty spaces where their careers, childcare responsibilities, and solid expectations about the future used to reside, China's congregational dancers have created a place where they can enjoy their remaining years with people of their choosing and doing what they wish. Though they have lost the security and guaranteed high status in old age that would have been afforded them had they been born a century earlier, they have also gained the freedom and resources to find alternative sources of support and meaning making. Armed with no blueprints for how to proceed and few resources other than camaraderie and a sense of adventure, they have somehow managed to find a new way of growing old that breaks previous molds. I did not expect to be amazed by the congregational dancers when I began this research; I did not expect to admire them. Yet during my time in Chengdu, I repeatedly found myself in awe of my interlocutors' displays of resilience, humor, and flexibility when confronted with unfamiliar or challenging situations. I am not sure that I can or will join a dance group when I retire, but I can only hope that I will have the same enthusiasm for life when I am their age.

I say that I am unsure whether I will join a group when I am older not only because I do not live in China, where this phenomenon is based, but also because this book has provided a snapshot into the experiences of a particular generation in a particular moment in time. I asked all my interlocutors—from congregational dancers to *shequ* officials to ordinary Chengdu residents—to weigh in on whether they thought the phenomenon will continue. Their responses varied: while some said that younger generations will definitely pick up congregational dancing as they get older, citing participants in their forties as evidence that dancers are not just retirees, others told me that this was a temporary phenomenon with an expiration date. Some of my younger Chinese friends and colleagues even burst into laughter at the question because the thought of themselves participating in congregational dance groups struck them as so absurd.

It is impossible to see the future, of course, but if I were forced to make a prediction, I would choose to side with those who say that congregational dancing will eventually run its course. However, I doubt that the phenomenon will disappear due to lack of interest from younger generations. People's interests change with age, and the same people who laugh now may be perfectly happy donning a fuchsia frock and dancing with a group of friends in thirty years. If congregational dance groups diminish in number or disappear from Chinese cities altogether, it will be because the conditions that currently make the phenomenon possible have changed.

Because I cannot travel into the future, I can perhaps best explain why I believe in the lasting impact of congregational dancing by telling a final story about a retired woman. In all the time I spent talking to retirees in Chengdu, I only met one person who decided to quit congregational dancing for reasons other than declining health or lack of time. She was a woman I called Auntie Liu (unrelated to the Auntie Liu who appears in an earlier chapter), and is a friend of one of my aunts by marriage. When Auntie Liu heard about my research project, she insisted on having me over to her house for tea, where she listened to me talk about my findings before sharing her own experiences with the congregational dancing phenomenon.

Auntie Liu is a retired high school teacher who was in a congregational dance group for seven years—2007 until 2014, until the group became, in her words, too caught up with competitions and *shequ* politics. She was in a group that met every morning at a small clearing in the riverside esplanade that runs through the south side of Chengdu. All was well until 2012, when city officials asked all dance groups who were using that section of the riverbank to move to a nearby park. The reason they gave was that dance groups were taking up too much space on the esplanade and disturbing other urban residents who wished to stroll or exercise. Auntie Liu's group moved to the park as requested, but park officials gave them a designated time allotment that limited their ability to come and go as they pleased. The group also had to abide by a noise ordinance that limited their music to a certain number of decibels. "In the summer," Auntie Liu told me, "you could barely hear the music over the sound of the cicadas." As if these regulations were not enough, local *shequ* officials soon recruited the group to perform in dance competitions, changing the focus and tone of the group's daily meetings. What was once a simple group of friends and acquaintances dancing together on the riverbank had transformed into an endless cycle of rehearsals, costume fittings, and meetings with *shequ* officials. Auntie Liu, who told me she joined the group to get some fresh air and to experience some artistry in her daily life, soon became frustrated and bored with the group's new status quo. Along with two other members, she decided to leave the group to pursue interests that were not subject to state interference.

Since then, Auntie Liu has tried various pastimes. First, she tried her hand at essay writing. She had some luck at first: she wrote a semi-fictional story based on events she had witnessed during a visit to distant relatives in a rural village and posted it online, where a junior editor at a literary magazine saw it and wanted to publish it. However, the magazine's editor in chief rejected the story just a few weeks before it was slated to appear in print. Apparently, the editor decided that the essay was politically incorrect because it contained vivid descriptions of poverty in the village. Auntie Liu was astonished and disappointed. She said the story had no political commentary; she had simply relayed some real-life events as they unfolded from her own perspective. The entire episode left a bad taste in Auntie Liu's mouth, and she gave up on writing shortly after. "I learned then that very few things are safe from politics," she said.

About one year before we met, Auntie Liu enrolled in a traditional Chinese ink-drawing class with a local teacher. She made a new group of friends in the class, and she now draws every day in her grown daughter's former bedroom, which she has converted into an art studio for herself. When I asked her why drawing was different from writing or dancing, she explained that it was different in at least two ways:

> First, unlike writing or dancing, you can keep your drawings to yourself. It's much more personal. You can't write something and just keep it in a pile, that's

not the point. Writings must be shared in order to achieve their potential. Same with dancing. You can't dance without an audience. Why do you think the *dama* are out in public all the time? But with drawings, you can draw, then put it away, then take it out to look again later, but you can get enjoyment from it without sharing it with anyone. Second, "they" [the state] don't understand art. Even if they looked, they would not be able to understand.

After this conversation, Auntie Liu took me back to her spare bedroom/art studio to show me some of her drawings. They were lovely examples of traditional Chinese landscapes and bird-and-flower paintings done in vibrant-colored inks on translucent papers and silks. They would not have been out of place in a museum shop or a store that catered to tourists. In other words, while it was clear that Auntie Liu had poured some part of herself into these drawings and found great personal meaning in them, it was not immediately apparent where in the drawings this meaning dwelled. Because she had chosen traditional subject matters and did not depart from conventional techniques and styles, the subjective dimensions of the pieces were obfuscated or concealed. Auntie Liu took great pride in this. Pointing to a painting of a hillside farmhouse done in shades of gray and green, she told me rather mysteriously, "You see a house; I see much more."

In her effort to imbue her life with meaning—to find what feels true and to say that truth out loud—Auntie Liu had retreated further and further into herself. The congregational dancing phenomenon had given her an outlet for meaning-making for some years, but its gradual integration into China's ideological landscape had forced her to seek out ever-narrower avenues elsewhere. Given her disdain for state-regulated pastimes and the high premium she places on individual expression, I thought that Auntie Liu had turned her back on congregational dancing entirely and for good. I was incredibly surprised, then, when she credited congregational dancing with turning her into who she was at the end of our conversation. She told me she had never considered personal expression or internal experience to be important aspects of life prior to retirement, and that she had learned to value these things during the course of her participation in her congregational dance group. "I left because it became too complicated," Auntie Liu explained. "But for me, dancing was the beginning of all of this. I wouldn't be drawing today if I hadn't danced back then."

Auntie Liu did not elaborate much beyond this, but I understood what she meant. She was no longer dancing, and yet her words echoed what many of my dance group interlocutors told me on a regular basis about what their participation in the phenomenon had given them: a sense of self, the confidence to prioritize their own needs, and the social support to validate their personal choices. Auntie Liu was no longer a congregational dancer, but her story showed me that the inner trappings of the phenomenon have the potential to reverberate beyond dancing itself, and that congregational dancing has the power to transform at least some aspects of Chinese society even if its duration is limited. It had certainly left a lasting impression on Auntie Liu. When I left her home, Auntie Liu gave me a small drawing of a bamboo grove on a stretched silk fan as a parting gift. "For you," she said as she handed it to me on my way out her front door. "Something to help you remember the *dama* by."

Since she was the only person I met who no longer participates in congregational dancing but was nevertheless transformed by her experience, it's possible that Auntie Liu is an anomaly. I suspect, however, that there are thousands or even millions more retirees throughout China whose worldviews and priorities have irrevocably changed because of their participation in the phenomenon. In dance groups all over the country, retired women are learning to embody a new kind of subjectivity that prioritizes personal experience while still considering the demands of other relationships. By focusing on something for the sake of personal enjoyment, and by sharing this enjoyment with people who share their interests, they are learning—however slowly—to develop avenues for individual expression and reshape their identities according to their own ideals. This is not the sort of skill that is taught by dance teachers or by online dance videos; it is not transmitted through model routines or official speeches at old age universities. It is an embodied knowledge that is cultivated in small increments over time; it emerges from countless conversations with friends about how to best grow old, from years of effort to balance family duties with emerging desires to prioritize one's own dreams, and from the realization that the *weidao* of being human—the substance that gives life its shape and its meaning—comes about via shared experiences but ultimately belongs to oneself alone.

That said, I would be quite surprised if these "dancing grannies" gathered to wage civil disobedience or antigovernment protests on behalf of their generation. Direct confrontation is simply not their style, and they have demonstrated that they can improvise their goals to better suit reality. For them, aging well, aging meaningfully, is not about having certainty about what lies ahead. They cannot count on that; it cannot be what defines their lives or what proves that they lived or aged well. Instead, it is about knowing everything is being done right now, in this moment, to squeeze as much joy out of life as it can hold. In the meantime, there is much to dance about.

References

Abrahams, Ray. 1999. "Friends and Networks as Survival Strategies in North-East Europe." In *The Anthropology of Friendship*, ed. Sandra Bell and Simon Coleman, 155–168. Oxford: Berg.
Anagnost, Ann. 1997. *National Past-Times: Narrative, Representation, and Power in Modern China*. Durham, NC: Duke University Press.
Angeloff, Tania, Marylène Lieber, and N. Jayaram. 2012. "Equality, Did You Say? Chinese Feminism after 30 Years of Reforms." *China Perspectives* 4 (92): 17–24.
Appleton, Simon, Lina Song, and Qingjie Xia. 2005. "Has China Crossed the River? The Evolution of Wage Structure in Urban China during Reform and Retrenchment." *Journal of Comparative Economics* 33 (4): 644–663.
Baker, Hugh D. R. 1979. *Chinese Family and Kinship*. London: Macmillan Education UK
Behar, Ruth, and Deborah A. Gordon. 1995. *Women Writing Culture*. Berkeley: University of California Press.
Béland, Daniel, and Ka Man Yu. 2004. "A Long Financial March: Pension Reform in China." *Journal of Social Policy* 33 (2): 267–288.
Blos, Peter. 1979. *The Adolescent Passage: Developmental Issues*. New York: International Universities Press.
Bray, David. 2005. *Social Space and Governance in Urban China: The Danwei System from Origins to Reform*. Stanford, CA: Stanford University Press.
Brownell, Susan. 1995. *Training the Body for China: Sports in the Moral Order of the People's Republic*. Chicago: University of Chicago Press.
Browning, Barbara. 1995. *Samba*. Bloomington: Indiana University Press.
Buckley, Chris. 2016. "'Dancing Granny' Is Shot, but Don't Expect the Music to Stop." *New York Times*, March 11, 2016. https://www.nytimes.com/2016/03/12/world/asia/china-dancing-square-grannies-shot.html.
Butler, Robert N. 2003. *Why Survive?: Being Old in America*. Baltimore: Johns Hopkins University Press.
Butler, Robert N., and Herbert P. Gleason. 1985. *Productive Aging: Enhancing Vitality in Later Life*. New York: Springer.

Carrier, James G. 1999. "People Who Can Be Friends: Selves and Social Relationships." In *The Anthropology of Friendship*, ed. Sandra Bell and Simon Coleman, 21–38. Oxford: Berg.

Carter, Liz. 2013. "China's Dancing Grannies Are Such a Nuisance They Are Being Pelted with 'Shit Bombs.'" *Foreign Policy* (blog), November 27, 2013. https://foreignpolicy.com/2013/11/27/chinas-dancing-grannies-are-such-a-nuisance-they-are-being-pelted-with-shit-bombs/.

Chawla, Devika. 2006. "Subjectivity and the 'Native' Ethnographer: Researcher Eligibility in an Ethnographic Study of Urban Indian Women in Hindu Arranged Marriages." *International Journal of Qualitative Methods* 5 (4): 13–29.

Chen, Feinian, Guangya Liu, and Christine A. Mair. 2011. "Intergenerational Ties in Context: Grandparents Caring for Grandchildren in China." *Social Forces* 90 (2): 571–594.

Chen, Nancy N. 2003. *Breathing Spaces: Qigong, Psychiatry, and Healing in China*. New York: Columbia University Press.

Chen, Sheying, and Elaina Y Chen. 2009. "Active Aging and China: Perspectives and Issues," In *Aging in China*, ed. Jason Powell and Ian Cook, 67–88. New York: Nova Science Publishers.

Chen, Wen-Cai, Si-Jing Chen, and Bao-Liang Zhong. 2022. "Sense of Alienation and Its Associations with Depressive Symptoms and Poor Sleep Quality in Older Adults Who Experienced the Lockdown in Wuhan, China, during the COVID-19 Pandemic." *Journal of Geriatric Psychiatry and Neurology* 35 (2): 215–222.

Chi, Sun [孙迟]. n.d. "Seniors Embrace the Digital Age through the Use of Smart Devices." Accessed August 2, 2023. https://www.chinadaily.com.cn/a/202303/11/WS640bceb5a31057c47ebb3b89.html.

Chin, Ai-li S., Maurice Freedman, and Joint Committee on Contemporary China Subcommittee on Research on Chinese Society. 1970. *Family and Kinship in Chinese Society*. Stanford, CA: Stanford University Press.

Chumley, Lily. 2016. *Creativity Class: Art School and Culture Work in Postsocialist China*. Princeton, NJ: University of Princeton Press.

Cliff, Tom. 2015. "Post-Socialist Aspirations in a Neo-Danwei." *China Journal* 73 (January): 132–157.

Clifford, James, and George E. Marcus. 1986. *Writing Culture: The Poetics and Politics of Ethnography: A School of American Research Advanced Seminar.*. Berkeley: University of California Press.

Cohen, Lawrence. 1998. *No Aging in India: Alzheimer's, the Bad Family, and Other Modern Things*. Berkeley: University of California Press.

Dante Alighieri. 1995a. *Dante's Inferno: The Indiana Critical Edition*. Translated by Mark Musa. Indiana Masterpiece Editions. Bloomington: Indiana University Press.

Davis, Deborah. 2000. *The Consumer Revolution in Urban China*. Berkeley: University of California Press.

Davis, Deborah, and Stevan Harrell, eds. 1993. *Chinese Families in the Post-Mao Era*. Berkeley: University of California Press.

Derleth, James, and Daniel R. Koldyk. 2004. "The Shequ Experiment: Grassroots Political Reform in Urban China." *Journal of Contemporary China* 13 (41): 747–777.

Dikötter, Frank. 2017. *The Cultural Revolution: A People's History, 1962–1976*. Reprint. London: Bloomsbury Press.

Domonoske, Camila. 2018. "69-Year-Old Dutch Man Seeks to Change His Legal Age to 49." NPR.org, November 8, 2018. https://www.npr.org/2018/11/08/665592537/69-year-old-dutch-man-seeks-to-change-his-legal-age-to-49.

Du, Fenglian, and Xiao-yuan Dong. 2009. "Why Do Women Have Longer Durations of Unemployment than Men in Post-Restructuring Urban China?" *Cambridge Journal of Economics* 33 (2): 233–252.

Dyson, Jane. 2010. "Friendship in Practice: Girls' Work in the Indian Himalayas." *American Ethnologist* 37 (3): 482–498.

"Elder in His 80s Pastes 'Plea for Adoption' on Street Corner" [八旬老人街头贴纸条'求收养']. N.d. Accessed March 20, 2018. https://m.sohu.com/a/211982901_255783?_f=m-index_important_news_11.

Fei, Xiaotong. 1992. *From the Soil: The Foundations of Chinese Society, A Translation of Fei Xiaotong's Xiangtu Zhongguo*. Berkeley: University of California Press.

Fong, Vanessa L. 2002. "China's One-Child Policy and the Empowerment of Urban Daughters." *American Anthropologist* 104 (4): 1098–1109.

———. 2004. *Only Hope: Coming of Age under China's One-Child Policy*. Stanford, CA: Stanford University Press.

Gladston, Paul. 2015. *Deconstructing Contemporary Chinese Art: Selected Critical Writings and Conversations, 2007–2014*. New York: Springer.

Goffman, Erving. 1959. *The Presentation of Self in Everyday Life*. New York: Doubleday Anchor Books.

Goh, Esther. 2011. *China's One-Child Policy and Multiple Caregiving*. London: Routledge.

Gratz, Tilo. 2004. "Friendship among Young Artisanal Gold Miners in Northern Benin (West Africa)." *Afrika Spectrum* 3 (1): 95–117.

Goldman, Andrea S. 2012. *Opera and the City: The Politics of Culture in Beijing, 1770–1900*. Stanford, CA: Stanford University Press.

Harwit, Eric. 2016. "WeChat: Social and Political Development of China's Dominant Messaging App." *Chinese Journal of Communication* 10 (3): 312–327.

Hayano, David M. 1979. "Auto-Ethnography: Paradigms, Problems, and Prospects." *Human Organization* 38 (1): 99–104.

Honig, Emily, and Xiaojian Zhao. 2015. "Sent-down Youth and Rural Economic Development in Maoist China." *China Quarterly* 222: 499–521.

Hsu, Becky Yang, and Richard Madsen, eds. 2019. *The Chinese Pursuit of Happiness: Anxieties, Hopes, and Moral Tensions in Everyday Life*. Berkeley: University of California Press.

Hsu, Francis L. K. 1967. *Under the Ancestors' Shadow: Kinship, Personality, and Social Mobility in Village China*. Garden City, NY: Anchor Books.

Hu, Jin, Peter-Josef Stauvermann, Surya Nepal, and Yuanhua Zhou. 2023. "Can the Policy of Increasing Retirement Age Raise Pension Revenue in China—A Case Study of Anhui Province." *International Journal of Environmental Research and Public Health* 20 (2): 1096.

Huang, Claudia. 2016. "'Dancing Grannies' in the Modern City: Consumption and Group Formation in Urban China." *Asian Anthropology* 15 (3): 225–241.

———. 2021. "Becoming Dama: The New Old Age in Urban China." *Journal of Aging Studies* 57 (June): 100928.

"Is Taking Care of Grandchildren the Destiny of All Older People in China?" [带孙子, 是中国老年人全部的宿命吗?]. N.d. Accessed September 23, 2019. https://known.ifeng.com/a/20180905/45152277_0.shtml.

Kanuha, Valli Kalei. 2000. "'Being' Native versus 'Going Native': Conducting Social Work Research as an Insider." *Social Work* 45 (5): 439–447.

Kaufman, Sharon R. 1986. *The Ageless Self: Sources of Meaning in Late Life*. Madison: University of Wisconsin Press.

Kawachi, Ichiro, and Lisa F. Berkman. 2001. "Social Ties and Mental Health." *Journal of Urban Health: Bulletin of the New York Academy of Medicine* 78 (3): 458–467.

Khan, Natasha. 2022. "Inside a Shanghai Mass Quarantine Center: No Showers, Lights on 24/7." *Wall Street Journal*, April 17, 2022. https://www.wsj.com/articles/inside-a-shanghai-mass-quarantine-center-no-showers-lights-on-24-7-11650187802.

Kipnis, Andrew. 2009. "Education and the Governing of Child-Centered Relatedness." In *Chinese Kinship: Contemporary Anthropological Perspectives*, ed. Susanne Brandstädter and Gonçalo D. Santos, 204–222. London: Routledge.

Kong, Nancy, Lars Osberg, and Weina Zhou. 2019. "The Shattered 'Iron Rice Bowl': Intergenerational Effects of Chinese State-Owned Enterprise Reform." *Journal of Health Economics* 67 (September): 102220.

Kuan, Teresa. 2015. *Love's Uncertainty: The Politics and Ethics of Child Rearing in Contemporary China*. Berkeley: University of California Press.

Lamb, Sarah. 2000. *White Saris and Sweet Mangoes: Aging, Gender, and Body in North India*.: California Digital Library UC Press E-Books Collection, 1982–2004 (Open Access). Berkeley: University of California Press.

———. 2009. *Aging and the Indian Diaspora: Cosmopolitan Families in India and Abroad*. Bloomington: Indiana University Press.

———. 2013. "Permanent Personhood or Meaningful Decline? Toward a Critical Anthropology of Successful Aging." *Journal of Aging Studies* 29 (April): 41–52.

Law, Wing-Wah, and Wai-Chung Ho. 2011. "Music Education in China: In Search of Social Harmony and Chinese Nationalism." *British Journal of Music Education* 28 (3): 371–388.

Lei, Guang. 2003. "Rural Taste, Urban Fashions: The Cultural Politics of Rural/Urban Difference in Contemporary China." *Positions: East Asia Cultures Critique* 11 (3): 613–646.

Lesko, Nancy. 2012. *Act Your Age!: A Cultural Construction of Adolescence*. 2nd ed. New York: Routledge.

Leung, Joe C. B. 1994. "Dismantling the 'Iron Rice Bowl': Welfare Reforms in the People's Republic of China." *Journal of Social Policy* 23 (3): 341–361.

Liebelt, C. 2016. "Manufacturing Beauty, Grooming Selves: The Creation of Femininities in the Global Economy—An Introduction." *Sociologus* 66 (1): 9–24.

Linders, Annulla. 2016. "Deconstructing Adolescence." Cham: Springer International Publishing.

Liu, Haoming. 2011. "Economic Reforms and Gender Inequality in Urban China." *Economic Development and Cultural Change* 59 (4): 839–876.

Liu, Jingyuan, Crystal Kwan, Jie Deng, and Yuxi Hu. 2022. "The Mental Health Impact of the COVID-19 Pandemic on Older Adults in China: A Systematic Review." *International Journal of Environmental Research and Public Health* 19 (21): 14362.

Liu, Xin. 2000. *In One's Own Shadow: An Ethnographic Account of the Condition of Post-Reform Rural China*. Berkeley: University of California Press.

———. 2002. *The Otherness of Self: A Genealogy of the Self in Contemporary China*. Ann Arbor: University of Michigan Press.

Luo, Baozhen, and Heying Zhan. 2012. "Filial Piety and Functional Support: Understanding Intergenerational Solidarity among Families with Migrated Children in Rural China." *Ageing International* 37 (1): 69–92.

Ma, Laurence J. C. 2006. "Social Space and Governance in Urban China: The Danwei System from Origins to Reform." *China Journal* 55: 176–179.

Mahler, Margaret S. 1977. *Separation–Individuation: Essays in Honor of Margaret S. Mahler.* Northvale, NJ: Jason Aronson.

Malaby, Thomas M. 2009. "Anthropology and Play: The Contours of Playful Experience." *New Literary History* 40 (1): 205–218.

McWilliams, Sally E. 2012. "'People Don't Attack You If You Dress Fancy': Consuming Femininity in Contemporary China." *Women's Studies Quarterly* 41 (1/2): 162–181.

Mead, Margaret. (1928) 1961. *Coming of Age in Samoa: A Psychological Study of Primitive Youth for Western Civilization.* New York: Morrow Quill.

Mor-Barak, Michál E., and Leonard S. Miller. 1991. "A Longitudinal Study of the Causal Relationship between Social Networks and Health of the Poor Frail Elderly." *Journal of Applied Gerontology* 10 (3): 293–310.

Morris, Andrew D. 2004. *Marrow of the Nation: A History of Sport and Physical Culture in Republican China.* Berkeley: University of California Press.

Narayan, Kirin. 1993. "How Native Is a 'Native' Anthropologist?" *American Anthropologist* 95 (3): 671–686.

"Our Country Is Enacting Legislation to Deal with the Noise Caused by Square Dancing and the Roar of Cars that 'Blow Up the Streets'" ["我国正立法应对广场舞噪声扰民、机动车轰鸣'炸街'"]. China News Service. December 17, 2021. https://www.chinanews.com.cn/gn/2021/12-17/9632023.shtml.

Palmer, David A. 2007. *Qigong Fever: Body, Science, and Utopia in China.* New York: Columbia University Press.

Parish, William L., and Martin King Whyte. 1978. *Village and Family in Contemporary China.* Chicago: University of Chicago Press.

Pitt-Rivers, Julian. 1973. "The Kith and the Kin." In *The Character of Kinship,* ed. Jack R. Goody, 89–105. Cambridge: Cambridge University Press.

Posen, Adam S. 2023. "The End of China's Economic Miracle." *Foreign Affairs,* August 2, 2023. https://www.foreignaffairs.com/china/end-china-economic-miracle-beijing-washington.

Powell, Jason L. 2012. "China and the Bio-Medicalization of Aging: Implications and Possibilities." In *Aging in China: Implications to Social Policy of a Changing Economic State,* edited by Sheying Chen and Jason L. Powell, 11–22. Boston: Springer.

Quillian, Lincoln, and Devah Pager. 2001. "Black Neighbors, Higher Crime? The Role of Racial Stereotypes in Evaluations of Neighborhood Crime." *American Journal of Sociology* 107 (3): 717–767.

Rofel, Lisa. 2007. *Desiring China: Experiments in Neoliberalism, Sexuality, and Public Culture.* Durham, NC: Duke University Press.

Rothschild, Viola. 2019. "China's Pension System Is Not Aging Well." *The Diplomat.* Accessed May 30, 2019. https://thediplomat.com/2019/03/chinas-pension-system-is-not-aging-well/.

Rowe, J. W., and R. L. Kahn. 1997. "Successful Aging." *Gerontologist* 37 (4): 433–440.

Ruan, Lotus, Masashi Crete-Nishihata, Jeffrey Knockel, Ruohan Xiong, and Jakub Dalek. 2020. "The Intermingling of State and Private Companies: Analysing Censorship of the 19th National Communist Party Congress on WeChat." *China Quarterly* 246 (June): 497–526.

Ruby, Jay, ed. 2016. *A Crack in the Mirror: Reflexive Perspectives in Anthropology.* Philadelphia: University of Pennsylvania Press.

Santos, Gonçalo D., and Stevan Harrell. 2016. *Transforming Patriarchy: Chinese Families in the Twenty-First Century.* Seattle: University of Washington Press.

Santos-Granero, Fernando. 2007. "Of Fear and Friendship: Amazonian Sociality beyond Kin-ship and Affinity." *Journal of the Royal Anthropological Institute* 13 (1): 1–18.

Shea, Jeanne L. 2005. "Sexual 'Liberation' and the Older Woman in Contemporary Mainland China." *Modern China* 31 (1): 115–147.

Shen, Liang, and Hong Fan. 2021. "Sport, Ideology and Nation-Building in the Early Years of the People's Republic of China." *International Journal of the History of Sport* 38 (17): 1774–1790.

Song, Shunfeng. 2003. "Policy Issues of China's Urban Unemployment." *Contemporary Economic Policy* 21 (2): 258–269.

Stanley-Becker, Isaac. 2018. "A 69-Year-Old Man Asks to Be Declared 49, Claiming Age Is as Fluid as Gender." *Washington Post*, November 8, 2018. https://www.washingtonpost.com/nation/2018/11/08/year-old-man-asks-be-declared-claiming-age-is-fluid-gender/.

Stevenson, Alexandra. "The World Tries to Move Beyond Covid. China May Stand in the Way." *New York Times*, May 13, 2022. https://www.nytimes.com/2022/05/13/business/china-zero-covid-xi.html.

Tang, Wenfang, and William L. Parish. 2000. *Chinese Urban Life under Reform: The Changing Social Contract.* Cambridge: Cambridge University Press.

Thomason, Erin. 2021. "United in Suffering." In *Chinese Families Upside Down*, ed. Yunxiang Yan, 76–102. Leiden, Netherlands: Brill Publishers.

Thurston, Anne F. 1984. "Victims of China's Cultural Revolution: The Invisible Wounds: Part I." *Pacific Affairs* 57 (4): 599–620.

"To Take or Not to Take a 'Grandchild Care Fee': Elders All Have Opinions for Their Adult Children" ["带孙费"到底该不该要 老人与儿女都有话说]. N.d. Accessed October 28, 2019. http://inews.ifeng.com/yidian/46075914/news.shtml?ch=ref_zbs_ydzx_news.

Tsuda, Takeyuki. 2015. "Is Native Anthropology Really Possible?" *Anthropology Today* 31 (3): 14–17.

Tu, Mingwei. 2016. "Chinese One-Child Families in the Age of Migration: Middle-Class Transnational Mobility, Ageing Parents, and the Changing Role of Filial Piety." *Journal of Chinese Sociology* 3 (1): 1–17.

Walder, Andrew G. 1983. "Organized Dependency and Cultures of Authority in Chinese Industry." *Journal of Asian Studies* 43 (1): 51–76.

Wang, Di. 2003. *Street Culture in Chengdu: Public Space, Urban Commoners, and Local Politics, 1870–1930.* Stanford, CA: Stanford University Press.

———. 2008. *Violence and Order on the Chengdu Plain: The Story of a Secret Brotherhood in Rural China, 1939–1949.* Stanford, CA: Stanford University Press.

———. 2018. *The Teahouse under Socialism.* Ithaca, NY: Cornell University Press.

Watson, Rubie S. 1986. "The Named and the Nameless: Gender and Person in Chinese Society." *American Ethnologist* 13 (4): 619–631.

Weller, Robert P. 1999. *Alternate Civilities: Democracy and Culture in China and Taiwan.* Boulder, CO: Westview Press.

Whyte, Martin King. 2012. "China's Post-Socialist Inequality." *Current History* 111 (746): 229–234.
Wilcox, Emily E. 2011. "The Dialectics of Virtuosity: Dance in the People's Republic of China, 1949–2009." PhD diss., University of California.
———. 2018a. "Dynamic Inheritance: Representative Works and the Authoring of Tradition in Chinese Dance." *Journal of Folklore Research* 55 (1): 77–111.
———. 2018b. *Revolutionary Bodies: Chinese Dance and the Socialist Legacy*. Berkeley: University of California Press.
Winner, Ellen. 1989. "How Can Chinese Children Draw so Well?" *Journal of Aesthetic Education* 23 (1): 41–63.
Wolf, Margery. 1972. *Women and the Family in Rural Taiwan*. Stanford, CA: Stanford University Press.
World Bank. 2018. World Bank. Accessed August 8, 2023. https://www.worldbank.org/en/country/china/overview.
World Health Organization (WHO). 2022. "Ageing and Health." Accessed March 7, 2023. https://www.who.int/news-room/fact-sheets/detail/ageing-and-health.
Xu, Jing. 2017. *The Good Child: Moral Development in a Chinese Preschool*. Stanford, CA: Stanford University Press.
Yan, Yunxiang. 1996. *The Flow of Gifts: Reciprocity and Social Networks in a Chinese Village*. Stanford, CA: Stanford University Press.
———. 2003. *Private Life under Socialism: Love, Intimacy, and Family Change in a Chinese Village, 1949–1999*. Stanford, CA: Stanford University Press.
———. 2009. *The Individualization of Chinese Society*. London School of Economics Monographs on Social Anthropology, v 77. New York: Berg.
———. 2016. "Intergenerational Intimacy and Descending Familism in Rural North China." *American Anthropologist* 118 (2): 244–257.
———. 2017. "Doing Personhood in Chinese Culture." *Cambridge Anthropology* 35 (2): 1–17.
Yang, Jie. 2011. "Nennu and Shunu: Gender, Body Politics, and the Beauty Economy in China." *Signs* 36 (2): 333–357.
Yang, Mayfair. 1994. *Gifts, Favors, and Banquets: The Art of Social Relationships in China*. Ithaca, NY: Cornell University Press.
Yurchak, Alexei. 2005. *Everything Was Forever, Until It Was No More: The Last Soviet Generation*. Princeton, NJ: Princeton University Press.
Zang, Li, and Aihwa Ong. 2008. *Privatizing China: Socialism from Afar*. Ithaca, NY: Cornell University Press.
Zhang, Hong. 2017. "Recalibrating Filial Piety: Realigning the Family, State, and Market Interests in China?" In *Transforming Patriarchy: Chinese Families in the Twenty-First Century*, ed. Gonçalo D. Santos and Stevan Harrell, 234–250. Seattle: University of Washington Press.
Zhang, Li. 2010. *In Search of Paradise: Middle-Class Living in a Chinese Metropolis*. Ithaca, NY: Cornell University Press.
Zhang, Yuanting, and Franklin W. Goza. 2006. "Who Will Care for the Elderly in China? A Review of the Problems Caused by China's One-Child Policy and Their Potential Solutions." *Journal of Aging Studies* 20 (2): 151–164.
Zhong, Xiaohui, and Minggang Peng. 2020. "The Grandmothers' Farewell to Childcare Provision under China's Two-Child Policy: Evidence from Guangzhou Middle-Class Families. *Social Inclusion* 8 (2): 36–46.

Zhou, Wuping, Lanyue Zhang, Ting Wang, Qiaosheng Li, and Weiyan Jian. 2022. "Influence of Social Distancing on Physical Activity among the Middle-Aged to Older Population: Evidence from the Nationally Representative Survey in China." *Frontiers in Public Health* 10. https://www.frontiersin.org/articles/10.3389/fpubh.2022.958189.

Zhu Haoyun, and Alan Walker. 2018. "Pension System Reform in China: Who Gets What Pensions?" *Social Policy Administration* 52: 1410–1424.

INDEX

active aging, 8, 103
adolescence, 8–9, 41

Beijing Dance Academy, 97–98, 105
Butler, Robert, 7
Browning, Barbara, 16

Chinese Communist Party
   revolution, 3, 43, 103
   role in regulating art and expression, 26, 55, 93, 96–109, 113
   state-society relations, 22–34, 43, 55, 115
Chumley, Lily, 109
Confucius, 42–44
consumer culture, 24–25, 50–53, 121
Cohen, Lawrence, 41
congregational dancing
   choreography, 4, 96–97, 104
   costumes and props, 27, 29, 101–103, 122
   disputes over noise, 28, 32–33, 95, 119, 122, 124
   government regulation of, 91–108, 111–114, 123
   groups and organization, 27–32, 54, 57, 60–62
   origins of, 26–27, 35–36
   rural areas, 106–108
COVID-19 pandemic, 116–119

dama
   attire and appearance, 46–51
   generational identity, 8–10, 73
   stereotypes of, 38–40
dance competitions, 31, 99–111, 124
danwei system, 25
Davis, Deborah, 25, 49, 55
demographic changes, 6–8, 34, 41–46, 52–53, 68, 120
Deng Xiaoping, 21, 23, 25, 43, 48
Dyson, Jane, 56

eldercare
   caring for elderly parents, 62, 85–87. *See also* intergenerational relations
   institutions, 75
   plans for, 77–90
exercise, 8, 17, 26–27, 112, 117

Fei Xiaotong, 24
filial piety
   changing understandings of, 62, 72
   in custom, 54–55, 58–59, 87
   in policy, 42–44, 66, 88–89
friendship
   anthropology of, 56
   as social safety net, 79–81

gender, 10–11, 40, 49–53
General Administration of Sports, 94–96, 98–99

Goffman, Erving, 45
Goldman, Andrea, 109
Great Proletarian Cultural Revolution
    experiences during, 3, 20, 26, 33, 78,
    impact on art culture, 43, 93, 99, 110, 116
grandparents, 2, 54–72, 84

Inferno (Dante), 40
insider anthropology, 15
intergenerational relations, 54–55, 83–84.
    See also grandparents

Kaufman, Sharon, 44

Lamb, Sarah, 8, 41
Liu, Xin, 45–46

Mahler, Margaret, 8
Malaby, Thomas, 90
Mao Zedong, 4, 21–23, 92–93, 99, 102
McWilliams, Sally, 50
Mead, Margaret, 41
medical care
    health insurance, 74–75
    retirees' concerns about, 81–83
Ministry of Culture, 94–96, 98–99, 110, 114

New Culture Movement, 43

old age universities, 15, 33–34, 60, 70, 116
one-child policy
    experiences of, 3, 21
    impact on intergenerational relations,
        24, 32, 53, 75–80, 84
    reform, 68–71
Ong, Aihwa, 4

Palmer, David, 26
play, 75–90
pensions, 55, 75, 79, 115, 120–121
population aging. *See* demographic changes

Ratelband, Emile, 52–53
retirement
    adjusting to, 35, 81, 84–85, 121
    compulsory age of, 10–11, 43, 77–78, 120
    hobbies, 33–35, 53, 123–126

Rofel, Lisa, 25, 49
Rowe, John and Robert Kahn, 7-.8 *See also*
    successful aging

sandwich generation, 54–55, 71 *See also*
    grandparents
self-expression
    in art, 93, 108–112
    in congregational dancing, 30, 91–92,
        99–106
    regulation of, 93–99, 112–114
senior benefits, 35, 38. *See also* pensions
Sichuanese dialect, 15, 75–76
Su Min, 1–3, 6
successful aging, 7–8
state-owned enterprise (SOE) reforms, 10,
    21, 23, 32–33, 77–78, 120

terms of address, 16, 44–45, 61
Thomason, Erin, 55
twelve model routines, 94–99

Wang, Di, 13
Watson, Rubie, 44
WeChat
    congregational dancers' use of, 31, 38, 51,
        60–62, 65, 76–78, 85,
    regulation of, 115–118
Weller, Robert, 113
Wilcox, Emily, 27, 105
Winner, Ellen, 108
Wolf, Margery, 44
World Bank, 19, 42
World Health Organization, 7

Xi Jinping, 119
Xinhua News Agency, 94

Yan, Yunxiang, 9, 24, 40, 44
Yan'an Forum on Literature and Art, 93
Yang, Jie, 50
Yangge Tao (folk dance routines), 97–98,
    102, 111
Yurchak, Alexei, 5

Zhang, Hong, 66
Zhang, Li, 4, 25

About the Author

CLAUDIA HUANG immigrated to the United States from China with her parents when she was eight years old. She received her PhD in anthropology from UCLA and is currently an assistant professor of human development at California State University, Long Beach. She lives in Southern California with her husband, son, and cat.